Complement-Mediated Hemolytic Anemias

Editor

ROBERT A. BRODSKY

HEMATOLOGY/ONCOLOGY CLINICS OF NORTH AMERICA

www.hemonc.theclinics.com

Consulting Editors
GEORGE P. CANELLOS
H. FRANKLIN BUNN

June 2015 • Volume 29 • Number 3

ELSEVIER

1600 John F. Kennedy Boulevard • Suite 1800 • Philadelphia, Pennsylvania, 19103-2899

http://www.theclinics.com

HEMATOLOGY/ONCOLOGY CLINICS OF NORTH AMERICA Volume 29, Number 3
June 2015 ISSN 0889-8588, ISBN 13: 978-0-323-38890-0

Editor: Jennifer Flynn-Briggs
Developmental Editor: Barbara Cohen-Kligerman

Hematology/Oncology Clinics (ISSN 0889-8588) is published bimonthly by Elsevier Inc., 360 Park Avenue South, New York, NY 10010-1710. Months of issue are February, April, June, August, October, and December. Business and Editorial Offices: 1600 John F. Kennedy Blvd., Ste. 1800, Philadelphia, PA 19103–2899. Customer Service Office: 3251 Riverport Lane, Maryland Heights, MO 63043. Periodicals postage paid at New York, NY and at additional mailing offices. Subscription prices are $385.00 per year (domestic individuals), $633.00 per year (domestic institutions), $190.00 per year (domestic students/residents), $440.00 per year (Canadian individuals), $783.00 per year (Canadian institutions) $520.00 per year (international individuals), $783.00 per year (international institutions), and $255.00 per year (international and Canadian students/residents). International air speed delivery is included in all *Clinics* subscription prices. All prices are subject to change without notice. **POSTMASTER:** Send address changes to *Hematology/Oncology Clinics of North America*, Elsevier Health Sciences Division, Subscription Customer Service, 3251 Riverport Lane, Maryland Heights, MO 63043. Customer Service (orders, claims, online, change of address): Elsevier Health Sciences Division, Subscription **Customer Service, 3251 Riverport Lane, Maryland Heights, MO 63043. Tel: 1-800-654-2452 (U.S. and Canada); 314-447-8871 (outside U.S. and Canada). Fax: 314-447-8029. E-mail: journalscustomerservice-usa@elsevier.com (for print support); journalsonlinesupport-usa@elsevier.com (for online support).**

Reprints. For copies of 100 or more, of articles in this publication, please contact the Commercial Reprints Department, Elsevier Inc., 360 Park Avenue South, New York, New York 10010-1710; Tel.: 212-633-3874, Fax: 212-633-3820, E-mail: reprints@elsevier.com.

Hematology/Oncology Clinics of North America is covered in *MEDLINE/PubMed (Index Medicus), EMBASE/ Excerpta Medica, and BIOSIS.*

Contributors

CONSULTING EDITORS

GEORGE P. CANELLOS, MD
William Rosenberg Professor of Medicine, Department of Medical Oncology, Dana-Farber Cancer Institute, Boston, Massachusetts

H. FRANKLIN BUNN, MD
Professor of Medicine, Division of Hematology, Brigham and Women's Hospital, Harvard Medical School, Boston, Massachusetts

EDITOR

ROBERT A. BRODSKY, MD
The Johns Hopkins Family Professor of Medicine and Oncology; Director, Division of Hematology, The Johns Hopkins University School of Medicine, Baltimore, Maryland

AUTHORS

SIGBJØRN BERENTSEN, MD, PhD
Department of Medicine, Haugesund Hospital, Haugesund, Norway

ROBERT A. BRODSKY, MD
The Johns Hopkins Family Professor of Medicine and Oncology; Director, Division of Hematology, The Johns Hopkins University School of Medicine, Baltimore, Maryland

AMY E. DEZERN, MD, MHS
Assistant Professor of Oncology and Hematology, Division of Hematologic Malignancies, Department of Oncology, The Bunting and Blaustein Cancer Research Building, Baltimore, Maryland

BRITTA HÖCHSMANN, MD
Institute of Transfusion Medicine, University of Ulm; Institute of Clinical Transfusion Medicine and Immunogenetics Ulm; German Red Cross Blood Transfusion Service, Baden-Württemberg-Hessen; University Hospital of Ulm, Ulm, Germany

LINDSAY SUSAN KEIR, BSc, MBChB, MRCPCH, PhD
Department of Molecular and Cell Biology, Research Associate, The Scripps Research Institute, La Jolla, California; Clinical Lecturer, Academic Renal Unit, University of Bristol, Bristol, United Kingdom

JOEL MOAKE, MD
Department of Bioengineering, Rice University, Houston, Texas

ALISON R. MOLITERNO, MD
Assistant Professor of Medicine, Division of Hematology, Department of Medicine, The Johns Hopkins University School of Medicine, Baltimore, Maryland

RAKHI NAIK, MD, MHS
Assistant Professor of Medicine, Division of Hematology, Department of Medicine, The Johns Hopkins University School of Medicine, Baltimore, Maryland

ULLA RANDEN, MD, PhD
Department of Pathology, Oslo University Hospital, Oslo, Norway

ANTONIO M. RISITANO, MD, PhD
Head of Bone Marrow Transplantation Clinical Unit and Assistant Professor, Hematology, Department of Clinical Medicine and Surgery, Federico II University of Naples, Naples, Italy

SARAH SARTAIN, MD
Department of Bioengineering, Rice University; Section of Hematology-Oncology, Department of Pediatrics, Texas Children's Cancer and Hematology Centers, Baylor College of Medicine, Houston, Texas

WILLIAM J. SAVAGE, MD, PhD
Department of Pathology, Brigham and Women's Hospital, Boston, Massachusetts

HUBERT SCHREZENMEIER, MD
Institute of Transfusion Medicine, University of Ulm; Institute of Clinical Transfusion Medicine and Immunogenetics Ulm; German Red Cross Blood Transfusion Service, Baden-Württemberg-Hessen; University Hospital of Ulm, Ulm, Germany

SATISH SHANBHAG, MBBS, MPH
Assistant Professor of Medicine and Oncology, Division of Hematology, Department of Medicine, The Johns Hopkins University School of Medicine, Baltimore, Maryland

DAIMON P. SIMMONS, MD, PhD
Department of Pathology, Brigham and Women's Hospital, Boston, Massachusetts

C. JOHN SPERATI, MD, MHS
Assistant Professor of Medicine, Division of Nephrology, Department of Medicine, The Johns Hopkins University School of Medicine, Baltimore, Maryland

JERRY SPIVAK, MD
Professor of Medicine and Oncology, Division of Hematology, Department of Medicine, The Johns Hopkins University School of Medicine, Baltimore, Maryland

GEIR E. TJØNNFJORD, MD, PhD
Department of Haematology, Oslo University Hospital, Institute of Clinical Medicine, University of Oslo, Oslo, Norway

STEPHEN TOMLINSON, PhD
Department of Microbiology and Immunology, Ralph H. Johnson Veterans Affairs Medical Center, Medical University of South Carolina, Charleston, South Carolina

NANCY TURNER, BA
Department of Bioengineering, Rice University, Houston, Texas

JUAN CARLOS VARELA, MD, PhD
Division of Hematology, Department of Medicine, Sidney Kimmel Comprehensive Cancer Center, The Johns Hopkins University School of Medicine, Baltimore, Maryland

Contents

> The complement system is an essential component of the immune sys-
> tem. It is a highly integrative system and has a number of functions,
> including host defense, removal of injured cells and debris, modulation
> of metabolic and regenerative processes, and regulation of adaptive
> immunity. Complement is activated via different pathways and it is regu-
> lated tightly by several mechanisms to prevent host injury. Imbalance
> between complement activation and regulation can manifest in disease
> and injury to self. This article provides an outline of complement activation
> pathways, regulatory mechanisms, and normal physiologic functions of
> the system.

> ABO incompatibility of red blood cells leads to brisk complement-
> mediated lysis, particularly in the setting of red cell transfusion. The ABO
> blood group is the most clinically significant blood group because of pre-
> formed immunoglobulin M (IgM) and IgG antibodies to ABO blood group
> antigens (isohemagglutinins) in everyone except group AB individuals. In
> addition to transfusion, ABO incompatibility can cause hemolysis in he-
> matopoietic and solid organ transplantation, hemolytic disease of the
> newborn, and intravenous immunoglobulin infusion. It is important to pre-
> vent ABO incompatibility when possible and to anticipate complications
> when ABO incompatibility is unavoidable.

> Warm autoimmune hemolytic anemia (AIHA) is defined as the destruction
> of circulating red blood cells (RBCs) in the setting of anti-RBC autoanti-
> bodies that optimally react at 37°C. The pathophysiology of disease in-
> volves phagocytosis of autoantibody-coated RBCs in the spleen and
> complement-mediated hemolysis. Thus far, treatment is aimed at
> decreasing autoantibody production with immunosuppression or reducing
> phagocytosis of affected cells in the spleen. The role of complement inhi-
> bitors in warm AIHA has not been explored. This article addresses the
> diagnosis, etiology, and treatment of warm AIHA and highlights the role
> of complement in disease pathology.

Cold antibody types account for about 25% of autoimmune hemolytic anemias. Primary chronic cold agglutinin disease (CAD) is characterized by a clonal lymphoproliferative disorder. Secondary cold agglutinin syndrome (CAS) complicates specific infections and malignancies. Hemolysis in CAD and CAS is mediated by the classical complement pathway and is predominantly extravascular. Not all patients require treatment. Successful CAD therapy targets the pathogenic B-cell clone. Complement modulation seems promising in both CAD and CAS. Further development and documentation are necessary before clinical use. We review options for possible complement-directed therapy.

Paroxysmal cold hemoglobinuria is a rare cause of autoimmune hemolytic anemia predominantly seen as an acute form in young children after viral illnesses and in a chronic form in some hematological malignancies and tertiary syphilis. It is a complement mediated intravascular hemolytic anemia associated with a biphasic antibody against the P antigen on red cells. The antibody attaches to red cells at colder temperatures and causes red cell lysis when blood recirculates to warmer parts of the body. Treatment is mainly supportive and with red cell transfusion, but immunosuppressive therapy may be effective in severe cases.

Paroxysmal nocturnal hemoglobinuria is manifests with a chronic hemolytic anemia from uncontrolled complement activation, a propensity for thrombosis and marrow failure. The hemolysis is largely mediated by the alternative pathway of complement. Clinical manifestations result from the lack of specific cell surface proteins, CD55 and CD59, on PNH cells. Complement inhibition by eculizumab leads to dramatic clinical improvement. While this therapeutic approach is effective, there is residual complement activity resulting from specific clinical scenarios as well as from upstream complement components that can account for suboptimal responses in some patients. Complement inhibition strategies are an area of active research.

The severe clinical symptoms of inherited CD59 deficiency confirm the importance of CD59 as essential complement regulatory protein for protection of cells against complement attack, in particular protection of hematopoietic cells and human neuronal tissue. Targeted complement inhibition might become a treatment option as suggested by a case report. The easy diagnostic approach by flow cytometry and the advent of a new treatment option should increase the awareness of this rare differential diagnosis and lead to further studies on their pathophysiology.

Nancy Turner, Sarah Sartain, and Joel Moake

> The molecular linkage between ultralarge (UL) von Willebrand factor (VWF) multimers and the alternative complement pathway (AP) has recently been described. Endothelial cell (EC)-secreted and anchored ULVWF multimers (in long stringlike structures) function as both hyperadhesive sites that initiate platelet adhesion and aggregation and activating surfaces for the AP. In vitro, the active form of C3, C3b binds to the EC-anchored ULVWF multimeric strings and initiates the assembly on the strings of C3 convertase (C3bBb) and C5 convertase (C3bBbC3b). In vivo, activation of the AP via this mechanism proceeds all the way to generation of terminal complement complexes (C5b-9).

Lindsay Susan Keir

> Shiga toxin associated hemolytic uremic syndrome (Stx HUS), a thrombotic microangiopathy, is the most common cause of pediatric acute kidney injury but has no direct treatment. A better understanding of disease pathogenesis may help identify new therapeutic targets. For this reason, the role of complement is being actively studied while eculizumab, the C5 monoclonal antibody, is being used to treat Stx HUS but with conflicting results. A randomized controlled trial would help properly evaluate its use in Stx HUS while more research is required to fully evaluate the role complement plays in the disease pathogenesis.

C. John Sperati and Alison R. Moliterno

> Thrombotic microangiopathies (TMA) such as atypical hemolytic uremic syndrome (aHUS) have evolved from rare, fulminant childhood afflictions to uncommon diseases with acute and chronic phases involving both children and adults. Breakthroughs in complement and coagulation regulation have allowed redefinition of specific entities despite substantial phenotypic mimicry. Reconciliation of phenotypes and delivery of life saving therapies require a multidisciplinary team of experts. The purpose of this review is to describe advances in the molecular pathophysiology of aHUS and to share the 2014 experience of the multidisciplinary Johns Hopkins TMA Registry in applying diagnostic assays, reporting disease associations, and genetic testing.

Antonio M. Risitano

> The availability of anticomplement therapies has been a major achievement for medicine in the last decade. Indeed, eculizumab has changed the treatment paradigm of paroxysmal nocturnal hemoglobinuria and

atypical hemolytic uremic syndrome and promises to do the same in several other human complement-mediated diseases. Nowadays, a 10-year experience has also taught us that there are some pitfalls that represent a challenge to improve the current anticomplement treatment. Most of these observations come from paroxysmal nocturnal hemoglobin-uria, where unmet clinical needs are emerging, triggering the attention of several investigators and pharmaceutical companies.

HEMATOLOGY/ONCOLOGY CLINICS OF NORTH AMERICA

ISSUE OF RELATED INTEREST

Clinics in Laboratory Medicine, March 2015 (Vol. 35, Issue 1)
Automated Hematology Analyzers: State of the Art
Carlo Brugnara and Alexander Kratz, *Editors*
Available at: http://www.labmed.theclinics.com/

THE CLINICS ARE AVAILABLE ONLINE!
Access your subscription at:
www.theclinics.com

Preface

Complement in Health and Disease

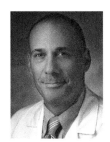

Robert A. Brodsky, MD
Editor

The complement system is a major effector of innate immunity. It consists of more than 40 serum and membrane proteins that are tightly regulated to protect the host from a variety of pathogens. Disruption of the balance between complement activation and regulation is central to the pathophysiology of many diseases. Over the past decade there has been remarkable progress in understanding the role of complement in a variety of hemolytic anemias. Moreover, novel pharmacologic inhibitors of the complement cascade are rapidly making their way into clinical medicine and having a dramatic impact on heretofore life-threatening hemolytic diseases. This issue covers complement regulation, outlines the major hemolytic diseases caused by activation of the complement system, and reviews current and future strategies for inhibiting the complement cascade.

Robert A. Brodsky, MD
Division of Hematology
Johns Hopkins University School of Medicine
720 Rutland Avenue
1025 Ross Research Building
Baltimore, MD 21205, USA

E-mail address:
brodsro@jhmi.edu

Hematol Oncol Clin N Am 29 (2015) xi
http://dx.doi.org/10.1016/j.hoc.2015.02.003
0889-8588/15/$ – see front matter © 2015 Published by Elsevier Inc.

Complement
An Overview for the Clinician

 CrossMark

Juan Carlos Varela, MD, PhD[a], Stephen Tomlinson, PhD[b],*

KEYWORDS

- Complement system • Complement activation • Complement regulation
- Complement function • Inflammation • Immune response

KEY POINTS

- The complement system is composed of over 50 interacting serum and membrane-bound proteins that provides an effective immune surveillance.
- Complement can be activated via 3 different pathways: the classical, lectin, and alternative pathways, which converge at the cleavage and activation of C3 with the subsequent generation of various biological effector molecules.
- Strict regulation of the complement system is mediated by a number of soluble and membrane-bound proteins to prevent damage to self.
- Complement plays a key role in a number of biological processes, including host defense, removal of injured cells and debris, modulation of metabolic and regenerative processes, and the regulation of adaptive immunity.
- Inappropriate complement activation and impaired regulation can lead to self-directed attack and contributes to various diseases and disease-related conditions.

The complement system is a major component of the innate immune system and it provides a powerful and effective mechanism to protect the host from pathogens. It was first described in the late 19th century as a heat-labile component of serum that "complemented" the effects of antibodies in the lysis of bacteria and red blood cells.[1–4] The term *complement* was coined by Paul Ehrlich in 1899.[5,6] We now know that the complement system is made up of some 50 serum and membrane proteins with tightly regulated proteolytic activation cascades that culminate in the production of effector molecules with multiple biological functions.[4–9] It has long been known that complement provides host surveillance and protection from microbes, and it is now

The authors have nothing to disclose.
[a] Division of Hematology, Department of Medicine, Sidney Kimmel Comprehensive Cancer Center, The Johns Hopkins University School of Medicine, Baltimore, MD, USA; [b] Department of Microbiology and Immunology, Ralph H. Johnson Veterans Affairs Medical Center, Medical University of South Carolina, Charleston, SC, USA
* Corresponding author.
E-mail address: tomlinss@musc.edu

Hematol Oncol Clin N Am 29 (2015) 409–427
http://dx.doi.org/10.1016/j.hoc.2015.02.001
0889-8588/15/$ – see front matter Published by Elsevier Inc.

clear that complement also plays important and diverse roles in several other physiologic and homeostatic functions, such as the clearance of dead and dying cells, developmental and regenerative processes, and the modulation of humoral and cell-mediated immune responses.[10] Furthermore, disruption of the balance between complement activation and complement regulation is involved in the pathogenesis of several diseases and disease states, ranging from traumatic injury and ischemia-related conditions, to autoimmune disease, to alloreactivity and transplant rejection. Complement is also implicated in tumor immune surveillance, and recently tumor-promoting functions of complement have also been described.[11,12]

Soluble complement proteins are synthesized primarily by hepatocytes, although significant amounts are also synthesized by monocytes, macrophages, and some epithelial cells in the gastrointestinal and urinary tracts.[5] Activation of complement is normally achieved via 3 different pathways: the classical, alternative, and lectin pathways. Each of these pathways is initiated by different stimuli (**Table 1**), but all lead to the cleavage and activation of the central complement protein C3, with the subsequent cleavage of C5 and generation of biological effector molecules. In addition to the 3 well-defined pathways of activation, there are also bypass mechanisms of activation, such as the direct proteolytic cleavage of C5.[13]

ACTIVATION OF THE COMPLEMENT SYSTEM
The Classical Pathway

The classical pathway is triggered by antibody-antigen immune complexes via C1q recognition of Fc domains in conformationally altered immunoglobulin (Ig)M or clustered IgG (**Fig. 1**). The interaction of C1q with Fc causes a conformational change within the C1q molecule and the subsequent cleavage and activation of the associated C1r and C1s serine proteases. Activated C1s then cleaves C4 and C2 into 2 large active fragments (C4b and C2a) and 2 small soluble inactive fragments (C4a and C2b). Cleavage of C4 exposes a reactive thioester within the C4b fragment, which results in covalent attachment of C4b to the activating surface. The binding of C2 to C4b and the subsequent cleavage of C2 result in the covalently attached classical pathway C3 convertase, C4bC2a (note that there is discrepancy in the literature in the designation of C2a vs C2b). This complex cleaves C3 into C3b (large) and C3a (small). Similar to C4b, C3b contains a reactive thioester that can become bound covalently to the activating surface, and that can initiate activation of the alternative pathway. If C3b binds to the C4bC2a complex, it forms to classical pathway C5 convertase (C4bC2aC3b) that cleaves C5 into C5b and C5a, with initiation of the terminal complement pathway.

Table 1	
Activation of the complement system	
Pathway	**Trigger for Activation**
Classical	Antibodies bound to bacteria, fungi, viruses, or tumor cells Immune complexes Apoptotic cells C-reactive protein Activated Factor XII
Alternative	Continuous hydrolysis of complement protein C3
Lectin	Microbes with terminal mannose groups
Other activators of complement	Thrombin Kallikrein

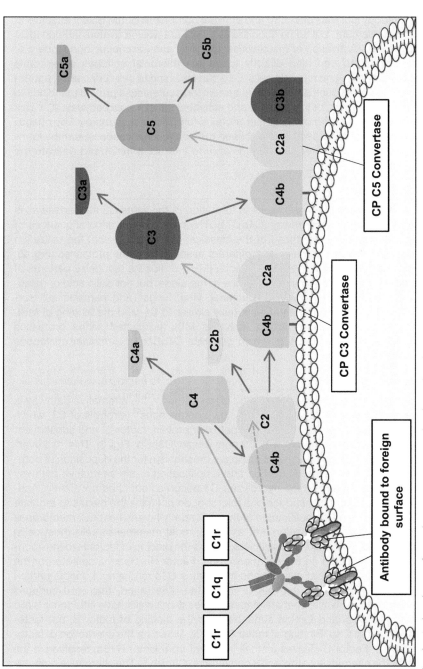

Fig. 1. The classical pathway of complement activation. The classical pathway is initiated by the binding of the C1 complex (C1q, C1r and C1s) to bound antibody. C1r activates C1s, which first cleaves C4 and then cleaves C2, leading to the formation of the classical pathway C3 convertase (C4bC2a). The C3 convertase subsequently cleaves C3 leading to the formation of the C5 convertase (C4bC2aC3b) and the release of the anaphylatoxin C3a. The C5 convertase then cleaves C5 into C5a and C5b. C5a is the most powerful of the anaphylatoxins and C5b is the first component of the terminal pathway of complement.

Both C3a and C5a are known as anaphylatoxins and are powerful biological effector molecules with diverse functions, including inflammation, modulation of adaptive immunity, and repair and regenerative processes.

Not all antibody isotypes bind C1q and activate complement. IgM is very effective at activating complement, but some subclasses of IgG are poor activators (human IgG4 and mouse IgG1). Activation of the classical pathway can also occur independent of antibodies, and C1q can bind directly to certain microbial epitopes or epitopes exposed on apoptotic and necrotic cells. C1q can also bind to cell surfaces via pattern recognition molecules such as C-reactive protein, an acute phase protein that binds to the surface of pathogens or injured cells and activates the classical pathway.[14–16] This process tags surfaces with complement proteins to facilitate their removal by phagocytes. An interaction can also occur between the coagulation cascade and the complement system, as activated factor XII is able to interact with C1 and activate the classical pathway.[17,18]

The Lectin Pathway

Activation of the lectin pathway results in formation of the same C3 convertase as is generated in the classical pathway (C4bC2a). The catalytic activation sequences of the lectin pathway resemble those of the classical pathway, but with the utilization of different recognition molecules and different associated serine proteases (**Fig. 2**). In the lectin pathway, mannose-binding lectin (MBL) or ficolins recognize patterns of carbohydrates such as N-acetylglucosamine or mannose, but not sialic acid or galactose,[6] which provides selectivity for bacterial, viral, fungal, and parasitic cell surfaces.[19,20] MBL is structurally and functionally similar to C1, and the binding of MBL (or ficolin) to a carbohydrate ligand activates MBL-associated serine proteases (MASP-1, MASP-2, and MASP-3), which generate C4bC2a in a manner analogous to that of the C1 complex.

The Alternative Pathway

In contrast with the classical pathway and lectin pathway, the alternative pathway is constitutively active and depends on the slow spontaneous hydrolysis of C3, which exposes a binding site for the alternative pathway protein, factor B, and subsequent generation of the alternative pathway C3 convertase (C3bBb; **Fig. 3**). This "tickover" process provides a primed and rapid response mechanism for the deposition of complement on foreign surfaces. Activation and amplification of the alternative pathway depend on the surface to which hydrolyzed C3 becomes attached covalently. Activating surfaces, such as the surface of a microbe, do not have the means to regulate further C3 activation and amplification of the cascade, whereas host cell membranes effectively inhibit further activation. For example, most mammalian cells (host cells) have high levels of sialic acid, and sialic acid favors the binding of factor H to the spontaneously deposited C3b on the cell membrane. Factor H acts as a cofactor for the serine esterase factor I, that cleaves and inactivates C3b rendering it unable participate further in complement activation.[4,21] On the other hand, microbial surfaces such as bacterial cell walls, viral envelopes, or yeast cell walls have little to no sialic acid. Thus, microbial and foreign surfaces favor the binding of factor B, not factor H, to the deposited C3b. Binding of factor B to C3b allows for the interaction of factor D with factor B. Factor D cleaves a small fragment from factor B (Ba) resulting in the formation of the alternative pathway C3 convertase, C3bBb.[22] The alternative pathway C3 convertase is stabilized by properdin, which extends the half-life of the convertase.[23] The alternative pathway C3 convertase subsequently cleaves more C3 molecules leading to the rapid generation of C3b, and this amplification loop also amplifies

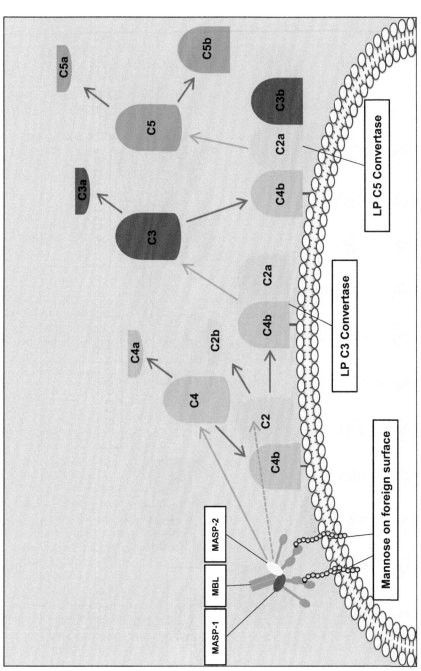

Fig. 2. The lectin pathway of complement activation. The steps in components and reaction in the lectin pathway are very similar to those in the classical pathway. The only differences are the initiation steps. The lectin pathway is initiated by binding of the complex of mannose-binding lectin (MBL) and the serine proteases MBL-associated proteases 1 and 2 (MASP-1 and MASP-2) to mannose groups on the surface of invading pathogens. Next, MASP-1 activates MASP-2, which acts like C1s in the classical pathway, and leads to the formation of the C3 convertase. The remaining steps are the same as in the classical pathway.

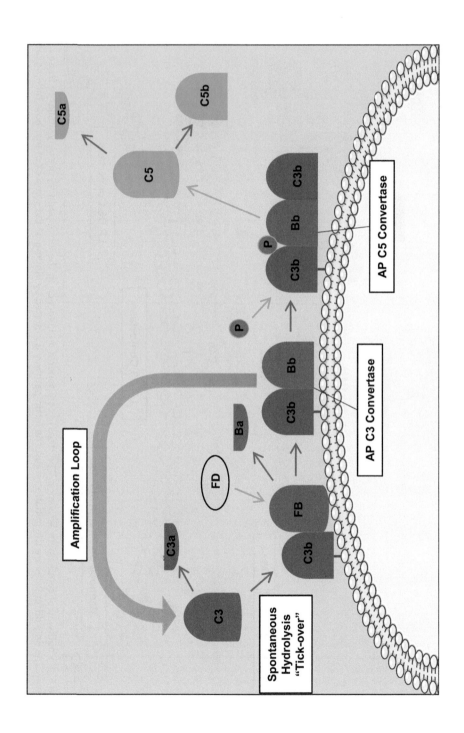

the generation of C3b produced via the classical pathway and lectin pathway. The binding and cleavage of an additional C3 molecule to C3bBb forms the alternative pathway C5 convertase, C3bBbC3b, with the same function as the classical pathway C5 convertase. The alternative pathway can also be activated by the binding of properdin to molecular patterns found on pathogens or injured cells and the subsequent recruitment of fluid phase C3b.[24]

Regardless of how complement is activated (classical, lectin, or alternative pathway), it has been estimated that the alternative pathway accounts for about 80% of generated complement activation products, and as such it is a major driver of inflammation.[25]

The Terminal Pathway of Complement

All 3 pathways of complement activation converge at the formation of the C3 and C5 convertases, the latter of which cleaves C5. Cleavage of C5 produces the anaphylatoxin C5a, and a larger C5b fragment that initiates the nonenzymatic terminal pathway of complement (**Fig. 4**).

The cleavage of C5 exposes a binding site on C5b for C6. The resulting C5b-6 complex then binds C7 to form C5b-7, and upon formation of this trimeric complex, amphipathic sites are exposed that allow insertion into lipid bilayers.[26–29] In the event that C7 fails to bind to C5b-6, the complex is released and in the presence of C7 is able to bind to other nearby membranes. However, membrane insertion is an inefficient process, and most of the complexes are inactivated in the fluid phase. The C5b-7 complex than binds C8, exposing hydrophobic sites that form a stronger association with lipid bilayers. Finally, C5b-8 binds C9, which then unfolds in the membrane, which exposes further C9 binding sites. Thus, C5b-8 binds and polymerizes several C9 molecules, the result of which is a cytolytic transmembrane pore known as the membrane attack complex (MAC; C5b-9$_n$).

Additional Pathways of Complement Activation

In addition to the classical, alternative, and lectin pathways, it is now known that the complement system can be activated via other means. The best described of such interactions is the crosstalk between the complement, coagulation and fibrinolysis pathways. As described, activated factor XII is able to activate the classical pathway of complement activation. Additionally, thrombin has been shown to both cleave C3[30,31] and also act as a C5 convertase, hence, bypassing the early pathways of complement activation.[13] It is also well-described that plasmin and kallikrein directly cleave C3 and its activation fragments.[18,31–33]

Relevant to the current discussion is recent data investigating complement activation in the pathophysiology of the thrombotic microangiopathies. Evidence suggests that thrombotic thrombocytopenic purpura, atypical hemolytic uremic syndrome,

Fig. 3. The alternative pathway of complement activation. The alternative pathway is initiated by the spontaneous hydrolysis of C3 and the deposition of C3b on the surface of activating surfaces (nonhost surfaces) and the release of C3a. Factor B (FB) binds to C3b and is subsequently cleaved by factor D (FD) leading to the formation of the alternative pathway C3 convertase (C3bBb). Properdin (P, *green*) then binds to the convertase to stabilize it. The C3 convertase cleaves C3 releasing more C3a and resulting in the formation of the alternative pathway C5 convertase (C3bBbC3b). The C5 convertase then cleaves C5 into C5a and C5b. C5a is most powerful of the anaphylatoxins and C5b is the first component of the terminal pathway of complement.

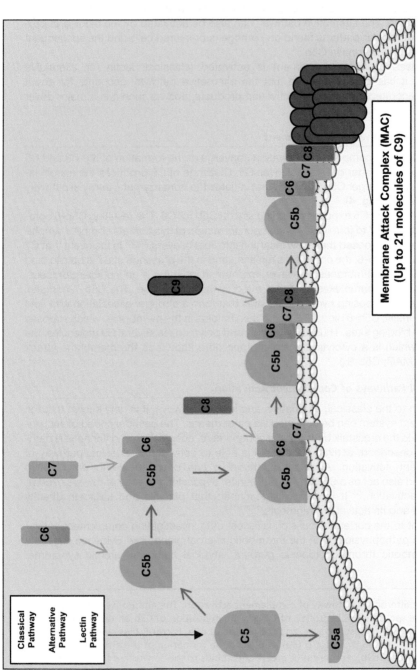

Fig. 4. The terminal pathway of complement. All 3 pathways of complement activation converge in the terminal pathway. The terminal pathway begins when C5b binds to C6. C7 then binds to the C5b–C6 complex and the newly formed C5b–C7 complex inserts into the target membrane. C8 subsequently binds to the C5b–C7 complex and creates a small pore in the target membrane. The final step in the terminal pathway is the binding of C9 molecules (≤21) to the C5b–C8 complex forming the membrane attack complex.

and typical Shiga toxin-induced hemolytic uremic syndrome are all diseases of aberrant complement activation.[34] It is well-known that atypical hemolytic uremic syndrome results from uncontrolled complement activation secondary to mutation in complement regulatory proteins.[35] However, until recently Shiga toxin-induced hemolytic uremic syndrome and thrombocytopenic purpura were not considered to be complement-mediated diseases. In thrombocytopenic purpura, current reports suggest widespread activation of complement as an important pathogenic mechanism.[36–38] In Shiga toxin-induced hemolytic uremic syndrome, it is thought that complement is activated via p-selectin, which is upregulated as a result of endothelial damage caused by Shiga toxin.[39,40]

REGULATION OF THE COMPLEMENT SYSTEM

Complement activation leads to the induction of a number of potent immunologic processes. This powerful effector system has the potential to do significant damage to the host if not kept in check, and it is therefore tightly regulated. A "builtin" mechanism of regulation for all complement pathways is that many of the intermediate activation products are very unstable and are inactivated spontaneously if they do not interact rapidly with other components of the cascade. In addition, there are several complement regulatory proteins expressed by the host that include both membrane-bound and fluid phase inhibitors. These inhibitors can be general, or can be activation pathway or terminal pathway specific. Before engaging in a discussion of the functions of individual complement inhibitors, it is pertinent to discuss the mechanisms that regulate the expression of complement inhibitors. Although the exact mechanisms leading to the modulation of complement inhibitor expression in vivo are not well understood, in vitro studies indicate that cytokines play a significant role. Several cytokines including interleukin-4, tumor necrosis factor-α, interferon-γ, interleukin-1β, and transforming growth factor-β have been shown to induce an increase in the expression of complement inhibitors on endothelial cells in vitro.[41–44] Complement inhibitors protect the host against collateral complement damage during episodes of complement activation (eg, inflammatory responses). Hence, there is interconnection between important players in an inflammatory response (ie, cytokines) and mechanisms leading to complement inhibitor expression. The following is a review of some important soluble and membrane-bound complement inhibitors.

Soluble Inhibitors of Complement

C1 inhibitor
The first step in the classical pathway is mediated by the C1 complex (C1q, C1r, and C1s), and the first step in the lectin pathway is mediated by MBL or a ficolin complex (MBL/ficolin, MASP-1, MASP-2, MASP-3). C1-inhibitor (C1-inh) inhibits C1r and C1s proteases of the classical pathway, and MASP-1 and MASP-2 proteases of the lectin pathway, with the result of preventing cleavage of C4 and C2.[45]

C4-binding protein and factor I
C4-binding protein (C4bp) binds to C4b and accelerates the decay of the classical pathway C3 convertase, and also serves as cofactor for the serine protease factor I. Factor I cleaves C4b into the inactive fragments C4c and C4d.[46,47] Factor I can also cleave and inactivate C3b. C4bp regulates the classical and lectin pathways, whereas factor I is involved in regulating the classical, alternative, and lectin pathways.

Factor H

Factor H is a plasma protein that regulates the alternative pathway both in the fluid phase and on cell surfaces. After binding to C3b, factor H functions by preventing the formation of, or causing the dissociation of, the alternative pathway C3 convertase. Factor H also serves as a cofactor for factor I, leading to the cleavage and inactivation of C3b and preventing further progress of the complement cascade.[48,49] Because the alternative pathway spontaneously activates on any surface and amplifies the other complement pathways, factor H provides an important regulatory mechanism to prevent host cell injury.

Mannose-binding lectin–associated protein of 44 kDa

The initial step in activation of the lectin pathway is the binding of MBL or ficolins to carbohydrate patterns and the subsequent cleavage of C4 and C2 by associated MASPs. An additional protein known as mannose-binding lectin–associated protein of 44 kDa (Map44 or MAP1) is also associated with the MBL/ficolin–MASP complex, and this nonproteolytic protein inhibits the lectin pathway by displacing the MASPs from MBL/ficolins and thus preventing C4 and C2 cleavage.[50–52]

Membrane-Bound Inhibitors of Complement

Complement receptor type 1

Complement receptor 1 (CR1 or CD35) is a glycoprotein expressed predominantly on blood cell types including erythrocytes and leukocytes.[53,54] It is a receptor for C3b and C4b, and one important function of CR1 is the removal of complement opsonized microbes or immune complexes via their transport to the liver or spleen. CR1 expressed on certain leukocytes can also facilitate phagocytosis of complement-opsonized cells. CR1 functions as a complement inhibitor by acting as a cofactor for factor I–mediated cleavage and inactivation of C3b and C4b, a mechanism analogous to the function of C4bp and factor H. In addition, CR1 can accelerate the decay of the C3 and C5 convertases.[55]

Membrane cofactor protein

Membrane cofactor protein (MCP) is a transmembrane protein that is associated mostly with control of the alternative pathway convertases, although it is reported to modulate the classical and lectin pathways as well.[56] It is expressed on most cell types, except erythrocytes. The complement regulatory functions of MCP are similar to those of CR1. Like CR1, MCP acts a cofactor for factor I in the cleavage and inactivation of C4b and C3b. However, unlike CR1, it does not promote the decay of the C3 or C5 convertases. MCP can also bind to C4b and C3b and block the formation of the C3 and C5 convertases. This protein has also been shown to downregulate T-helper type 1 immune responses.[57]

Decay accelerating factor

Decay accelerating factor (DAF) is attached to the cell membrane via a glycosyl-phosphatidylinositol anchor and it is expressed in most tissues.[58] It inhibits the formation of both the classical pathway and alternative pathway C3 convertases, as well as accelerates their decay. Additionally, an alternatively spliced DAF cDNA has been reported and it is thought to encode for a secreted form of the protein.[59]

CD59

Like DAF, CD59 is a glycosyl-phosphatidylinositol–anchored protein. It is expressed abundantly and widely.[53] CD59 is the only well-characterized inhibitor of the terminal pathway, and it functions by binding to C8 and C9 in the assembling MAC, thus interfering with C9 binding, polymerization, and pore formation.[60,61]

Additional Pathways of Complement Regulation

As described, there is significant crosstalk between the complement, coagulation, and fibrinolysis cascades. This crosstalk not only leads to complement activation, but it can also lead to complement regulation. For example, thrombomodulin, an important component of the fibrinolytic pathway, can accelerate the factor I–mediated inactivation of C3b.[62] In addition, thrombomodulin also enhances the thrombin-mediated activation of procarboxypeptidase B, an inhibitor of the fibrinolytic pathway, resulting in inactivation of C3a and C5a.[62]

FUNCTIONS OF THE COMPLEMENT SYSTEM

The complement system has diverse physiologic functions, and is additionally intertwined with several other biological networks, thus expanding the universe of its activity. Herein, we discuss only some of the more well-known and better-documented functions of complement.

Protection of the Host Against Infection

As an essential component of the innate immune system, complement is a first line of defense against many invading pathogens. Initial infection by microorganisms such as bacteria, viruses, and parasites can differently activate any complement pathway, depending on the composition of the microbe surface. This activation is triggered by components such as lipopolysaccharides, peptidoglycans, and certain carbohydrates (eg, mannose). The classical pathway and lectin pathway can also be triggered by natural IgM antibodies that recognize non–self-microbial antigens.[63–65] In addition, the classical pathway can be activated if pathogen-specific antibodies are also present in the host. Complement activation can lead to formation of the MAC on the surface of the invading microorganism, but MAC-mediated cytolysis is not effective against most microorganisms. For example, with regard to bacterial infection, deficiency in one of the terminal complement proteins leads to increased susceptibility to Neisserial infection only.

A more important complement-dependent mechanism of host defense involves complement receptor–dependent phagocytosis of complement-opsonized pathogens. As described, factor I cleaves C3 into iC3b and C3f. Factor I further cleaves iC3b into C3c and C3dg. Subsequently, serum proteases cleave C3dg into C3g and C3d. These C3 activation products are covalently bound to activating surfaces and thus can opsonize microbes. Although these C3 fragments are unable to participate further in complement activation, they can bind to complement receptors on immune effectors cells and mediate phagocytosis of microorganisms. Complement-dependent phagocytosis is mediated primarily by complement receptors 3 and 4 (CR3 and CR4; **Table 2**). CR3 is a member of the β2 integrin family and it is a promiscuous receptor as it binds to iC3b, ICAM-1, LPS, fibrinogen, factor X, and some carbohydrates.[66] CR3 is expressed on monocytes, macrophages, neutrophils, natural killer cells, follicular dendritic cells, and subsets of T cells. CR4 belongs to the same family as CR3, and its ligands and tissue distribution are similar to that of CR3. CR3 is recognized as being the more important mediator of phagocytosis as determined by studies of patients with a deficiency in β2 integrins.[67,68]

Another complement mechanism that contributes to host defense is the induction of an inflammatory response. The complement fragments C3a and C5a are

Table 2
Distribution of complement receptors

Cell Type	CR1 C3b, C4b	CR2 C3d, C3dg, iC3b	CR3 iC3b	CR4 iC3b	C3aR C3a	C5aR C5a	C1qR C1q
Erythrocytes	X						
Platelets						X	X
Neutrophils	X		X	X	X	X	
Monocytes	X		X	X		X	
Macrophages	X		X	X		X	X
Eosinophils	X						
Basophils						X	
Mast cells						X	
Dendritic cells	X	X					
B cells	X	X					X
T cells	X	X	X	X	X	X	X
Natural killer cells			X	X			

anaphylatoxins and have varied and powerful effects in mediating inflammation. By interacting with their respective receptors, C3a and C5a mediate inflammation by variously increasing vascular permeability, inducing smooth muscle contraction, and the recruitment and activation of immune cells. They can also modulate the adaptive immune response to infectious agents. With regard to infection, C5a is generally considered the more potent of the anaphylatoxins at mediating inflammatory processes. The receptor for C5a is expressed on mast cells, basophils, neutrophils, monocytes, macrophages, endothelial cells, smooth muscle cells, and lymphocytes. In addition to causing degranulation of basophils and mast cells, C5a is a strong chemotactic agent for neutrophils, eosinophils, basophils, and monocytes.[69,70] C5a also plays an important role in the function of neutrophils and macrophages because it primes these phagocytic cells for enhanced functional responses.[71]

Immune Homeostasis and Disposal of Waste

The clearance of immune complexes and the clearance of dead and dying cells are important functions of complement. Binding of antibody to soluble antigen leads to the formation of immune complexes. These complexes become coated with C3b and subsequently bind to CR1 receptors on erythrocytes. Erythrocytes then carry the immune complexes to the liver and spleen where they are destroyed.[72] The failure to clear immune complexes results in their tissue deposition and complement activation, leading to inflammation and tissue injury. Complement also plays an important role in the clearance of apoptotic and injured cells. Apoptotic cells express neoepitopes on their surface that are recognized by natural circulating IgM antibodies. These antibodies activate both the classical pathway and lectin pathway, leading to complement opsonization of the apoptotic cell and complement-receptor–mediated phagocytosis. C1q can also bind directly to apoptotic cells, thus activating the classical pathway. The importance of this clearance process and of the role of complement is demonstrated by the fact that deficiency in certain complement proteins is strongly linked with the development of autoimmune disease.[21,73]

Tissue Repair, Regeneration, and Development

Few organs are able to regenerate in adult mammals, with the liver being a notable exception. Preclinical studies into the mechanism of hepatic regeneration have demonstrated an essential role for C3a and C5a in priming the hepatocyte proliferative response after injury or resection. This occurs via the effect of C3a/5a receptor signaling on cytokine and transcription factor expression.[74,75] Complement (principally C3a and C5a) has also been implicated in the regeneration of bone, cardiac muscle, and skeletal muscle, as well as stem cell engraftment (reviewed in[76–78]). Additionally, several groups have reported that complement also plays an important role in several key processes in the central nervous system.[77–79] Although the early consensus was that complement had mainly neurodegenerative and deleterious effects in the central nervous system, it is now apparent that complement is also involved in neuron regeneration, synapse formation, and neuroprotection. Particularly interesting is the finding that C1q and C3 opsonins play an essential role in synaptic pruning and neuron remodeling during development, which seems to occur via a mechanism analogous to that for immune homeostasis and apoptotic cell clearance.[80]

Bridging of the Innate and Adaptive Immune Responses

Role of complement in humoral immune responses

The complement system is not only an essential component of innate immunity, but also an important player in the induction of adaptive immune responses.[4,7,21,81,82] The role of complement in humoral immunity is well characterized and it is mediated via complement receptor 2 (CR2). CR2 is expressed primarily on B-cells, follicular dendritic cells, and certain T-cell subsets. Binding of complement (C3d)-opsonized antigen to CR2 on B cells reduces the threshold required for B-cell activation.[83,84] In addition, complement aids in the localization of antigen to FDCs within lymphoid follicles, promotes the development of B-cell memory and it can also enhance avidity maturation and class switching.[7,82,85–88]

Role of complement in cell-mediated immune responses

Complement can modulate all 3 phases of T-cell immune responses (ie, inductor phase, effector phase and contraction phase),[82,89–91] and plays an important role during cognate interactions between antigen-presenting cells and T cells. Signaling via costimulatory molecules (CD28, CD80, CD86, CD154 and CD40) results in (1) secretion of C3, factor B, factor D, and C5, (2) upregulation of the surface expression of C3a and C5a receptors (C3aR and C5aR), and (3) downregulation of surface expression of the complement inhibitor CD55 (DAF).[92–95] These changes in complement protein expression occur in both antigen-presenting cells and T cells, and via the local production of C3a and C5a results in autocrine and paracrine stimulation of the engaged antigen-presenting cells and T cells via C3aR and C5aR.[92–94] The role of complement in the effector phase of T-cell immunity has been shown in preclinical models showing that lack of C3 or C5aR leads to impaired $CD4^+$ and $CD8^+$ T-cell responses against viruses.[96–98] A role for complement in the contraction phase has also been demonstrated; concurrent crosslinking of the TCR and CD46 (MCP) on T cells leads to the development of regulatory T cells in vitro.[89,99] Recently, it has been shown that human T cells can process C3 to C3a and C3b intracellularly by cathepsin L cleavage, resulting in complement-dependent autocrine stimulation of T cells. Intracelluarly generated C3a was found to be required for T-cell survival, and after T-cell stimulation, induced the autocrine production of proinflammatory cytokines.[100] Finally, C3a and C5a receptor signaling can inhibit both natural and induced T-regulatory cell function, thereby further modulating the overall strength of a T-cell immune response.[101,102]

Depending on the context of complement activation and regulation, these effects of complement on the shaping of an adaptive immune response not only impacts immunity to infection, but also autoimmunity, alloimmunity and tumor immunity.

REFERENCES

1. Carroll MC, Fischer MB. Complement and the immune response. Curr Opin Immunol 1997;9:64–9.
2. Bordet J, Gengou O. Sur l'existence de substances sensibilisatrices dans la plupart des serum antimicrobiens. Ann Inst Pasteur 1901;15:289–302.
3. Metschnikoff E. Sur la lutte des cellule de l'organisme contre l'invasion des microbes. Ann Inst Pasteur 1887;1:321.
4. Walport MJ. Complement. First of two parts. N Engl J Med 2001;344:1058–66.
5. Goldsby R, Kindt T, Osborne BA, et al. Immunology. New York: Freeman and Company; 2003.
6. Paul W. Fundamental immunology. Philadelphia: Lippincott, Williams and Wilkins; 2003.
7. Carroll MC. The complement system in regulation of adaptive immunity. Nat Immunol 2004;5:981–6.
8. Rus H, Cudrici C, Niculescu F. The role of the complement system in innate immunity. Immunol Res 2005;33:103–12.
9. Kemper C, Pangburn MK, Fishelson Z. Complement nomenclature 2014. Mol Immunol 2014;61:56–8.
10. Ricklin D, Hajishengallis G, Yang K, et al. Complement: a key system for immune surveillance and homeostasis. Nat Immunol 2010;11:785–97.
11. Stover C. Dual role of complement in tumour growth and metastasis (Review). Int J Mol Med 2010;25:307–13.
12. Markiewski MM, DeAngelis RA, Benencia F, et al. Modulation of the antitumor immune response by complement. Nat Immunol 2008;9:1225–35.
13. Huber-Lang M, Sarma JV, Zetoune FS, et al. Generation of C5a in the absence of C3: a new complement activation pathway. Nat Med 2006;12:682–7.
14. Mold C, Gewurz H, Du Clos TW, et al. Regulation of complement activation by C-reactive protein. Immunopharmacology 1999;42:23–30.
15. Mold C, Du Clos TW, Nakayama S, et al. C-reactive protein reactivity with complement and effects on phagocytosis. Ann N Y Acad Sci 1982;389:251–62.
16. Gewurz H, Mold C, Siegel J, et al. C-reactive protein and the acute phase response. Adv Intern Med 1982;27:345–72.
17. Ghebrehiwet B, Silverberg M, Kaplan AP. Activation of the classical pathway of complement by Hageman factor fragment. J Exp Med 1981;153:665–76.
18. Rittirsch D, Flierl MA, Ward PA. Harmful molecular mechanisms in sepsis. Nat Rev Immunol 2008;8:776–87.
19. Iobst ST, Wormald MR, Weis WI, et al. Binding of sugar ligands to Ca(2+)-dependent animal lectins. I. Analysis of mannose binding by site-directed mutagenesis and NMR. J Biol Chem 1994;269:15505–11.
20. Iobst ST, Drickamer K. Binding of sugar ligands to Ca(2+)-dependent animal lectins. II. Generation of high-affinity galactose binding by site-directed mutagenesis. J Biol Chem 1994;269:15512–9.
21. Walport MJ. Complement. Second of two parts. N Engl J Med 2001;344:1140–4.
22. Volanakis JE, Narayana SV. Complement factor D, a novel serine protease. Protein Sci 1996;5:553–64.

23. Chapitis J, Lepow IH. Multiple sedimenting species of properdin in human serum and interaction of purified properdin with the third component of complement. J Exp Med 1976;143:241–57.
24. Cortes C, Ohtola JA, Saggu G, et al. Local release of properdin in the cellular microenvironment: role in pattern recognition and amplification of the alternative pathway of complement. Front Immunol 2012;3:412.
25. Harboe M, Mollnes TE. The alternative complement pathway revisited. J Cell Mol Med 2008;12:1074–84.
26. Podack ER, Kolb WP, Muller-Eberhard HJ. The C5b-9 complex: subunit composition of the classical and alternative pathway-generated complex. J Immunol 1976;116:1431–4.
27. Podack ER, Biesecker G, Müller-Eberhard HJ. Membrane attack complex of complement: generation of high-affinity phospholipid binding sites by fusion of five hydrophilic plasma proteins. Proc Natl Acad Sci U S A 1979;76:897–901.
28. Preissner KT, Podack ER, Müller-Eberhard HJ. The membrane attack complex of complement: relation of C7 to the metastable membrane binding site of the intermediate complex C5b-7. J Immunol 1985;135:445–51.
29. Podack ER, Müller-Eberhard HJ. Binding of desoxycholate, phosphatidylcholine vesicles, lipoprotein and of the S-protein to complexes of terminal complement components. J Immunol 1978;121:1025–30.
30. Clark A, Weymann A, Hartman E, et al. Evidence for non-traditional activation of complement factor C3 during murine liver regeneration. Mol Immunol 2008;45:3125–32.
31. Amara U, Flierl MA, Rittirsch D, et al. Molecular intercommunication between the complement and coagulation systems. J Immunol 2010;185:5628–36.
32. Thoman ML, Meuth JL, Morgan EL, et al. C3d-K, a kallikrein cleavage fragment of iC3b is a potent inhibitor of cellular proliferation. J Immunol 1984;133:2629–33.
33. Goldberger G, Thomas ML, Tack BF, et al. NH2-terminal structure and cleavage of guinea pig pro-C3, the precursor of the third complement component. J Biol Chem 1981;256:12617–9.
34. Noris M, Mescia F, Remuzzi G. STEC-HUS, atypical HUS and TTP are all diseases of complement activation. Nat Rev Nephrol 2012;8:622–33.
35. Noris M, Remuzzi G. Atypical hemolytic-uremic syndrome. N Engl J Med 2009;361:1676–87.
36. Ruiz-Torres MP, Casiraghi F, Galbusera M, et al. Complement activation: the missing link between ADAMTS-13 deficiency and microvascular thrombosis of thrombotic microangiopathies. Thromb Haemost 2005;93:443–52.
37. Réti M, Farkas P, Csuka D, et al. Complement activation in thrombotic thrombocytopenic purpura. J Thromb Haemost 2012;10:791–8.
38. Chapin J, Weksler B, Magro C, et al. Eculizumab in the treatment of refractory idiopathic thrombotic thrombocytopenic purpura. Br J Haematol 2012;157:772–4.
39. Morigi M, Galbusera M, Gastoldi S, et al. Alternative pathway activation of complement by Shiga toxin promotes exuberant C3a formation that triggers microvascular thrombosis. J Immunol 2011;187:172–80.
40. Del Conde I, Crúz MA, Zhang H, et al. Platelet activation leads to activation and propagation of the complement system. J Exp Med 2005;201:871–9.
41. Mason JC, Lidington EA, Ahmad SR, et al. bFGF and VEGF synergistically enhance endothelial cytoprotection via decay-accelerating factor induction. Am J Physiol Cell Physiol 2002;282:C578–87.

42. Mason JC, Yarwood H, Sugars K, et al. Induction of decay-accelerating factor by cytokines or the membrane-attack complex protects vascular endothelial cells against complement deposition. Blood 1999;94:1673–82.

43. Kawano M. Complement regulatory proteins and autoimmunity. Arch Immunol Ther Exp (Warsz) 2000;48:367–72.

44. Moutabarrik A, Nakanishi I, Namiki M, et al. Cytokine-mediated regulation of the surface expression of complement regulatory proteins, CD46(MCP), CD55(DAF), and CD59 on human vascular endothelial cells. Lymphokine Cytokine Res 1993;12:167–72.

45. Kirschfink M, Nürnberger W. C1 inhibitor in anti-inflammatory therapy: from animal experiment to clinical application. Mol Immunol 1999;36:225–32.

46. Blom AM, Kask L, Dahlbäck B. CCP1-4 of the C4b-binding protein alpha-chain are required for factor I mediated cleavage of complement factor C3b. Mol Immunol 2003;39:547–56.

47. Sim RB, Laich A. Serine proteases of the complement system. Biochem Soc Trans 2000;28:545–50.

48. Liszewski MK, Farries TC, Lublin DM, et al. Control of the complement system. Adv Immunol 1996;61:201–83.

49. Pangburn MK, Schreiber RD, Müller-Eberhard HJ. Human complement C3b inactivator: isolation, characterization, and demonstration of an absolute requirement for the serum protein beta1H for cleavage of C3b and C4b in solution. J Exp Med 1977;146:257–70.

50. Banda NK, Mehta G, Kjaer TR, et al. Essential role for the lectin pathway in collagen antibody-induced arthritis revealed through use of adenovirus programming complement inhibitor MAp44 expression. J Immunol 2014;193: 2455–68.

51. Pavlov VI, Skjoedt MO, Siow Tan Y, et al. Endogenous and natural complement inhibitor attenuates myocardial injury and arterial thrombogenesis. Circulation 2012;126:2227–35.

52. Degn SE, Hansen AG, Steffensen R, et al. MAp44, a human protein associated with pattern recognition molecules of the complement system and regulating the lectin pathway of complement activation. J Immunol 2009;183:7371–8.

53. Miwa T, Song WC. Membrane complement regulatory proteins: insight from animal studies and relevance to human diseases. Int Immunopharmacol 2001;1: 445–59.

54. Ahearn JM, Fearon DT. Structure and function of the complement receptors, CR1 (CD35) and CR2 (CD21). Adv Immunol 1989;46:183–219.

55. Iida K, Nussenzweig V. Functional properties of membrane-associated complement receptor CR1. J Immunol 1983;130:1876–80.

56. Kojima A, Iwata K, Seya T, et al. Membrane cofactor protein (CD46) protects cells predominantly from alternative complement pathway-mediated C3-fragment deposition and cytolysis. J Immunol 1993;151:1519–27.

57. Yamamoto H, Fara AF, Dasgupta P, et al. CD46: the "multitasker" of complement proteins. Int J Biochem Cell Biol 2013;45:2808–20.

58. Lublin DM, Atkinson JP. Decay-accelerating factor: biochemistry, molecular biology, and function. Annu Rev Immunol 1989;7:35–58.

59. Caras IW, Davitz MA, Rhee L, et al. Cloning of decay-accelerating factor suggests novel use of splicing to generate two proteins. Nature 1987;325:545–9.

60. Meri S, Morgan BP, Davies A, et al. Human protectin (CD59), an 18,000-20,000 MW complement lysis restricting factor, inhibits C5b-8 catalysed insertion of C9 into lipid bilayers. Immunology 1990;71:1–9.

61. Rollins SA, Sims PJ. The complement-inhibitory activity of CD59 resides in its capacity to block incorporation of C9 into membrane C5b-9. J Immunol 1990; 144:3478–83.
62. Delvaeye M, Noris M, De Vriese A, et al. Thrombomodulin mutations in atypical hemolytic-uremic syndrome. N Engl J Med 2009;361:345–57.
63. Baumgarth N, Herman OC, Jager GC, et al. Innate and acquired humoral immunities to influenza virus are mediated by distinct arms of the immune system. Proc Natl Acad Sci U S A 1999;96:2250–5.
64. Boes M, Prodeus AP, Schmidt T, et al. A critical role of natural immunoglobulin M in immediate defense against systemic bacterial infection. J Exp Med 1998;188: 2381–6.
65. Zhang M, Takahashi K, Alicot EM, et al. Activation of the lectin pathway by natural IgM in a model of ischemia/reperfusion injury. J Immunol 2006;177:4727–34.
66. Ehlers MR. CR3: a general purpose adhesion-recognition receptor essential for innate immunity. Microbes Infect 2000;2:289–94.
67. Coxon A, Rieu P, Barkalow FJ, et al. A novel role for the beta 2 integrin CD11b/CD18 in neutrophil apoptosis: a homeostatic mechanism in inflammation. Immunity 1996;5:653–66.
68. Hogg N, Stewart MP, Scarth SL, et al. A novel leukocyte adhesion deficiency caused by expressed but nonfunctional beta2 integrins Mac-1 and LFA-1. J Clin Invest 1999;103:97–106.
69. Fernandez HN, Henson PM, Otani A, et al. Chemotactic response to human C3a and C5a anaphylatoxins. I. Evaluation of C3a and C5a leukotaxis in vitro and under stimulated in vivo conditions. J Immunol 1978;120:109–15.
70. Morita E, Schröder JM, Christophers E. Differential sensitivities of purified human eosinophils and neutrophils to defined chemotaxins. Scand J Immunol 1989;29:709–16.
71. Ward PA. The dark side of C5a in sepsis. Nat Rev Immunol 2004;4:133–42.
72. Schifferli JA, Ng YC, Peters DK. The role of complement and its receptor in the elimination of immune complexes. N Engl J Med 1986;315:488–95.
73. Korb LC, Ahearn JM. C1q binds directly and specifically to surface blebs of apoptotic human keratinocytes: complement deficiency and systemic lupus erythematosus revisited. J Immunol 1997;158:4525–8.
74. Strey CW, Markiewski M, Mastellos D, et al. The proinflammatory mediators C3a and C5a are essential for liver regeneration. J Exp Med 2003;198:913–23.
75. He S, Atkinson C, Qiao F, et al. A complement-dependent balance between hepatic ischemia/reperfusion injury and liver regeneration in mice. J Clin Invest 2009;119:2304–16.
76. Phieler J, Garcia-Martin R, Lambris JD, et al. The role of the complement system in metabolic organs and metabolic diseases. Semin Immunol 2013;25:47–53.
77. Rutkowski MJ, Sughrue ME, Kane AJ, et al. Complement and the central nervous system: emerging roles in development, protection and regeneration. Immunol Cell Biol 2010;88:781–6.
78. Mastellos DC, Deangelis RA, Lambris JD. Complement-triggered pathways orchestrate regenerative responses throughout phylogenesis. Semin Immunol 2013;25:29–38.
79. Stephan AH, Barres BA, Stevens B. The complement system: an unexpected role in synaptic pruning during development and disease. Annu Rev Neurosci 2012;35:369–89.
80. Perry VH, O'Connor V. C1q: the perfect complement for a synaptic feast? Nat Rev Neurosci 2008;9:807–11.

81. Toapanta FR, Ross TM. Complement-mediated activation of the adaptive immune responses: role of C3d in linking the innate and adaptive immunity. Immunol Res 2006;36:197–210.

82. Kemper C, Atkinson JP. T-cell regulation: with complements from innate immunity. Nat Rev Immunol 2007;7:9–18.

83. Carter RH, Fearon DT. CD19: lowering the threshold for antigen receptor stimulation of B lymphocytes. Science 1992;256:105–7.

84. Dempsey PW, Allison ME, Akkaraju S, et al. C3d of complement as a molecular adjuvant: bridging innate and acquired immunity. Science 1996;271:348–50.

85. Fang Y, Xu C, Fu YX, et al. Expression of complement receptors 1 and 2 on follicular dendritic cells is necessary for the generation of a strong antigen-specific IgG response. J Immunol 1998;160:5273–9.

86. Carroll MC. The complement system in B cell regulation. Mol Immunol 2004;41: 141–6.

87. Molina H, Holers VM, Li B, et al. Markedly impaired humoral immune response in mice deficient in complement receptors 1 and 2. Proc Natl Acad Sci U S A 1996; 93:3357–61.

88. Test ST, Mitsuyoshi J, Connolly CC, et al. Increased immunogenicity and induction of class switching by conjugation of complement C3d to pneumococcal serotype 14 capsular polysaccharide. Infect Immun 2001;69:3031–40.

89. Kemper C, Chan AC, Green JM, et al. Activation of human CD4+ cells with CD3 and CD46 induces a T-regulatory cell 1 phenotype. Nature 2003;421:388–92.

90. Morgan BP, Marchbank KJ, Longhi MP, et al. Complement: central to innate immunity and bridging to adaptive responses. Immunol Lett 2005;97:171–9.

91. Longhi MP, Harris CL, Morgan BP, et al. Holding T cells in check–a new role for complement regulators? Trends Immunol 2006;27:102–8.

92. Lalli PN, Strainic MG, Yang M, et al. Locally produced C5a binds to T cell-expressed C5aR to enhance effector T-cell expansion by limiting antigen-induced apoptosis. Blood 2008;112:1759–66.

93. Strainic MG, Liu J, Huang D, et al. Locally produced complement fragments C5a and C3a provide both costimulatory and survival signals to naive CD4+ T cells. Immunity 2008;28:425–35.

94. Heeger PS, Lalli PN, Lin F, et al. Decay-accelerating factor modulates induction of T cell immunity. J Exp Med 2005;201:1523–30.

95. Liu J, Miwa T, Hilliard B, et al. The complement inhibitory protein DAF (CD55) suppresses T cell immunity in vivo. J Exp Med 2005;201:567–77.

96. Kopf M, Abel B, Gallimore A, et al. Complement component C3 promotes T-cell priming and lung migration to control acute influenza virus infection. Nat Med 2002;8:373–8.

97. Suresh M, Molina H, Salvato MS, et al. Complement component 3 is required for optimal expansion of CD8 T cells during a systemic viral infection. J Immunol 2003;170:788–94.

98. Kim AH, Dimitriou ID, Holland MC, et al. Complement C5a receptor is essential for the optimal generation of antiviral CD8+ T cell responses. J Immunol 2004; 173:2524–9.

99. Grossman WJ, Verbsky JW, Barchet W, et al. Human T regulatory cells can use the perforin pathway to cause autologous target cell death. Immunity 2004;21: 589–601.

100. Liszewski MK, Kolev M, Le Friec G, et al. Intracellular complement activation sustains T cell homeostasis and mediates effector differentiation. Immunity 2013;39:1143–57.

101. Strainic MG, Shevach EM, An F, et al. Absence of signaling into CD4+ cells via C3aR and C5aR enables autoinductive TGF-β1 signaling and induction of Foxp3+ regulatory T cells. Nat Immunol 2013;14:162–71.
102. Kwan W, van der Touw W, Paz-Artal E, et al. Signaling through C5a receptor and C3a receptor diminishes function of murine natural regulatory T cells. J Exp Med 2013;210:257–68.

Hemolysis from ABO Incompatibility

Daimon P. Simmons, MD, PhD, William J. Savage, MD, PhD*

KEYWORDS

- ABO blood group • ABH antigens • Isohemagglutinins • Complement • Hemolysis
- Major incompatibility • Minor incompatibility

KEY POINTS

- ABH antigens are the major antigens of the ABO blood group and are expressed on the cell surface in many tissues, including red blood cells.
- Most individuals express preformed immunoglobulin M (IgM) and IgG antibodies that bind to A and/or B antigens and cause hemolysis, largely through complement activation.
- Clinical situations involving ABO incompatible hemolysis include transfusion, hemolytic disease of the newborn, hematopoietic stem cell transplantation, solid organ transplantation, and intravenous immunoglobulin infusion.
- ABO incompatibility cannot always be avoided. An understanding of when and how ABO incompatible hemolysis occurs minimizes the incidence and adverse effects.

HISTORY

History provides several examples of the consequences of transfusing incompatible blood. The first report of a transfusion reaction was in the seventeenth century after transfusing humans with cow blood.[1] Centuries later, research in animals revealed that interspecies transfusions were more likely to result in fatal reactions,[2] and transfusions with human blood were attempted instead. Transfusions for severe obstetric hemorrhage were occasionally successful,[3,4] likely because of small transfusion volumes and serendipitous ABO compatibility.

In 1900, Landsteiner identified the ABO blood groups through agglutination testing.[5] This identification was possible because non-group O individuals make immunoglobulin M (IgM) and IgG antibodies that react with foreign A and/or B molecules expressed on erythrocyte cell membrane proteins. The clinical significance of Landsteiner's

The authors have nothing to disclose.
Department of Pathology, Brigham and Women's Hospital, 75 Francis Street, Boston, MA 02115, USA
* Corresponding author.
E-mail address: wjsavage@partners.org

Hematol Oncol Clin N Am 29 (2015) 429–443
http://dx.doi.org/10.1016/j.hoc.2015.01.003
0889-8588/15/$ – see front matter © 2015 Elsevier Inc. All rights reserved.

discovery is underscored by his receipt of the Nobel Prize in Physiology or Medicine in 1930. With the knowledge of the ABO blood group, transfusion services were established during World War I[6] and grew through the American Red Cross during World War II.[7]

Major and Minor ABO Incompatibility

Hemolytic reactions can occur either by transfusion of incompatible cells into a person with preformed antibodies (major incompatibility, **Fig. 1**) or by transfusion of antibodies into an incompatible recipient (minor incompatibility, **Fig. 2**).

ABO Testing

Blood banks test the ABO type of all blood donors and recipients. Forward typing to determine red cell antigen expression is performed by mixing antibodies against A and B separately with red blood cells. Antigen expression is indicated by erythrocyte agglutination after the addition of a specific antibody (**Fig. 3**). Reverse typing is performed by observing agglutination of reagent red cells to indicate the presence of antibody in plasma. Testing is performed manually in tubes (see **Fig. 3**) or in automated assays (**Fig. 4**). Complete ABO typing includes congruent forward and reverse typing.

Although these methods are reliable, ABO typing inconsistencies can arise. A and B expression can be lost in the setting of leukemia.[8] An acquired B phenotype occurs in the rare situation in which N-acetylgalactosamine (A substance) is converted into galactose (B substance) because of bacterial enzymatic changes in vivo.[9]

Recipient Type	Donor Type
O	A
	B
	AB
A	B
	AB
B	A
	AB

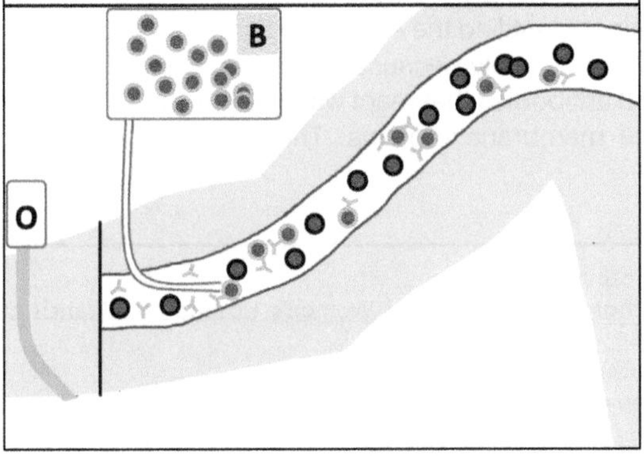

Fig. 1. Major ABO incompatibility. Transfusion of erythrocytes expressing B antigen into a type O patient with anti-B antibodies.

Recipient Type	Donor Type
AB	O
	A
	B
A	O
	B
B	O
	A

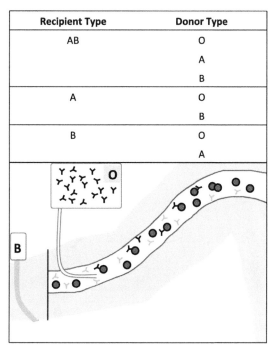

Fig. 2. Minor ABO incompatibility. Transfusion of plasma containing anti-B antibodies into a type B patient.

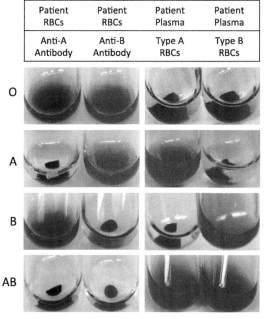

Patient RBCs	Patient RBCs	Patient Plasma	Patient Plasma
Anti-A Antibody	Anti-B Antibody	Type A RBCs	Type B RBCs

Fig. 3. Examples of tube agglutination assays for forward and reverse typing in individuals with each blood type. The extremes of 0 (soluble erythrocytes) and 4+ agglutination (a cell pellet) are demonstrated. Note that anti-A reagent is blue and anti-B reagent is yellow. RBCs, red blood cells.

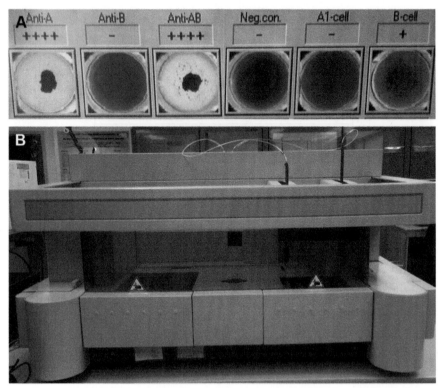

Fig. 4. An example of blood typing in a type A individual (with additional data on Rh excluded) (*A*) performed on an automated platform (*B*).

ABO ANTIGEN EXPRESSION AND BIOCHEMISTRY
ABO Antigen Structure

Only humans and higher apes express ABH antigens on red blood cells.[10] ABH antigens are also expressed in epithelial cells of the skin and mucosa as well as vascular endothelial cells and solid organ endothelium[11] in most vertebrates, including humans.

The ABO blood group comprises specific polysaccharide motifs on glycoproteins that are expressed at around 1 million antigens per erythrocyte.[12] The A and B groups represent a difference in the selection of a sugar molecule added to the H antigen, whereas the O group results from the absence of A or B sugars. The H antigen is formed by FUT1 enzymes adding fucose to glycoproteins,[13,14] resulting in a Fuc(α1-2)Gal(β1-3)GlcNAc(β1-R) motif (**Fig. 5**).[15] Individuals lacking the FUT1 enzyme have the Bombay phenotype and do not express the H antigen.[16] These individuals are incompatible with all ABO blood groups.

A small group of enzymes modifies polysaccharides to produce the ABH antigens, and minor changes in these enzymes cause significant changes in substrate specificity and activity. A and B antigens are produced through modification of the H antigen by glycosyltransferase enzymes (see **Fig. 5**) with substrate specificity for N-acetylgalactose (A antigen) or galactose (B antigen). Nucleotide changes in the DNA coding sequence determine whether the transferase will produce the A or B antigen. Other changes can either inactivate the protein or prevent translation entirely, resulting in the O phenotype.[17]

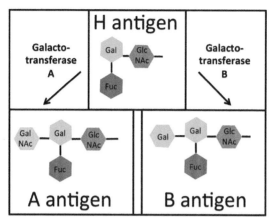

Fig. 5. The A and B antigens are created by the addition of sugar molecules to the H antigen by glycosyltransferase enzymes.

Other nucleotide changes affect the activity of glycosyltransferase, creating subgroups of A and B. The A_1 blood type is the most common subtype of A and expresses the A antigen at high levels on erythrocytes. In the A_2 blood type, a single nucleotide deletion leads to the extension of the protein by 21 amino acids[18] resulting in a functional protein with decreased activity. Thus, individuals with the A_2 phenotype have 10-fold lower levels of the A antigen than A_1 individuals.[19]

Epidemiology

The ABO blood group is present in different frequencies in populations around the world. Although type O is most common worldwide, type A is expressed fairly widely in African and European populations, whereas type B is more common in Asian populations (**Fig. 6**).[20]

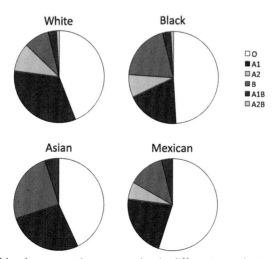

Fig. 6. The ABO blood group antigen expression in different populations.

PATHOPHYSIOLOGY

Initial exposure to an antigen is conventionally required for humoral antibody responses. Repeat exposure is necessary to drive antibody class switching and memory responses. This requirement is true for many blood group antigens, but most individuals express preformed antibodies to foreign ABH antigens without prior transfusion or pregnancy. These antibodies drive complement-mediated intravascular hemolysis during the first transfusion with ABO incompatible blood.

Natural ABO Antibodies

People spontaneously produce antibodies that recognize foreign ABH antigens. These natural antibodies neutralize viruses that express ABH antigens[21] and tend to be nonspecific with low affinity and auto-reactivity.[22,23] The most abundant ABO antibodies are low-affinity IgM molecules that cross-react with multiple antigens.[24,25] Antibody titers against A or B antigens are 6 to 10-fold higher in people who do not express those antigens (eg, type O individuals).[26] IgG antibodies are also produced against foreign A or B molecules.[27]

Natural antibody responses to foreign ABH molecules are enhanced by exposure to environmental microbes. Bacteria such as E. coli express a variety of polysaccharides[28] including some homologous to ABH antigens.[29] Total immunoglobulin levels are two-fold to three-fold lower in germ-free animals than normal ones,[30] and anti-B titers are undetectable in germ-free animals.[31] In humans, oral intake[32,33] or IV injection[34] of microbes that express ABH antigens drives antibody titers up to one hundred-fold higher. Humans naturally produce antibodies that cross-react with diverse pathogens, and coexistence with microbes drives higher titer IgM and IgG antibodies.

Complement Fixation and Red Blood Cell Lysis

When ABO-incompatible red blood cells are transfused, circulating antibodies bind to the ABH antigens and fix complement, resulting in hemolysis (see the article by Varela and Tomlinson elsewhere in this issue for more details). The proportion of ABO-incompatible erythrocytes that are hemolyzed depends on IgM titers.[35] Hemolysis occurs in the vasculature, liver, and spleen within minutes, followed by a second phase in which monocytes phagocytose erythrocytes coated with IgG, C3b, and C3d.[35,36]

An IgM pentamer is sufficient to fix complement, whereas different IgG subclasses have different efficiencies to fix complement and require at least 2 IgG molecules bound closely together.[37] ABH antigens are expressed at high density so antibody binding drives rapid complement fixation and formation of membrane attack complexes through the classical pathway. C5a generated through complement activation upregulates tissue factor expression on endothelial and immune cells, leading to diffuse intravascular coagulation. The complement cascade alters phospholipids on cell surfaces and creates a surface favorable to thrombosis.[38]

Intravascular hemolysis causes release of noxious intracellular products such as potassium and hemoglobin. Free hemoglobin is bound by haptoglobin and cleared by phagocytes. The system can be overwhelmed and cause hemoglobinemia (and subsequent hemoglobinuria), which depletes nitric oxide and causes endothelial dysfunction. At high levels, hemoglobinemia causes acute renal failure.[39] The release of intracellular contents through hemolysis and activation of inflammatory and coagulation pathways can be life threatening.

SETTINGS OF ABO INCOMPATIBLE REACTIONS

Although ABO-incompatible reactions are classically seen in the setting of mismatched red blood cell transfusion, major and minor ABO incompatibility may occur in a variety of different settings (**Box 1**).

Red Blood Cell Transfusion

Several different studies have identified the rate of ABO-incompatible red blood cell transfusions.[40–42] It is estimated that this occurs in as many as 1 in 38,000 transfusions,[42] which is significant given that 13 million red cell transfusions are given in the United States annually.

Hemolytic Disease of the Fetus and Newborn

Incompatibility of a mother and fetus can cause fetal hemolysis. Historically, the most common cause of hemolytic disease of the fetus and newborn (HDN) was Rh(D) incompatibility. ABO incompatibility is protective against Rh(D)-mediated HDN,[43,44] likely because of lysis of incompatible red cells before adaptive responses to the Rh(D) antigen can be initiated.[43] Now that prophylaxis is common for Rh(D)-incompatible pregnancies, ABO incompatibility is the most common cause of HDN.[45] Approximately 15% to 25% of babies are ABO incompatible with their mothers, but only approximately 1% have significant HDN[45] because IgM does not cross the placenta into fetal circulation. Additionally, because fetal erythrocytes express low levels of ABH antigens, hemolysis is rarely severe. HDN risk is highest when the mother has high titer IgG antibodies.[46] Phototherapy is typically sufficient for treatment.[45]

Platelet Transfusion

Platelets express ABH antigens; major ABO-incompatible platelet transfusion results in 20% lower posttransfusion platelet count increments, a difference that does not increase bleeding risk.[47,48] Few hospitals require ABO matching of platelets.[49]

The minor incompatibility of isohemagglutinins carried in the platelet-rich plasma is of greater concern because of the risk of hemolytic transfusion reactions. This risk is often tempered by the fact that isohemagglutinins also bind to epithelial cells.[50] Some institutions measure ABO antibody titers in platelet products before transfusion.[49] Hemolysis from minor incompatible platelet transfusion is generally related to the incompatible isohemagglutinin titer.[33,50,51]

Box 1
Settings of ABO incompatibility

- Incompatible red blood cell transfusion
- Mismatched platelets or plasma
- Hemolytic disease of newborn
- Hematopoietic stem cell transplant
- Solid organ transplant
- Intravenous immunoglobulin

Hematopoietic Stem Cell Transplant

When performing ABO-incompatible hematopoietic stem cell transplant (HSCT), both major and minor ABO incompatibility need to be considered.[52] ABO-incompatible HSCTs are performed in up to one-half of transplant centers. The data regarding effects of ABO incompatibility on survival are variable.[53–56]

Major incompatible HSCT is possible because hematopoietic stem cells do not express ABH antigens.[57] Major incompatible hemolysis may occur when a significant number of ABO-incompatible erythrocytes hemolyze during graft infusion. Management strategies include erythrocyte reduction of the graft and plasmapheresis to reduce the titer ABO antibodies in the recipient.[52] Major incompatibility may delay donor erythropoiesis.[58–60]

B lymphocytes are transplanted in HSCT and can produce isohemagglutinins. This situation is referred to as *passenger lymphocyte syndrome* and typically begins 1 to 2 weeks after graft infusion.[58] Passenger lymphocyte syndrome is characterized by delayed hemolysis of recipient red blood cells and significant hemolytic anemia.[61] These reactions typically resolve after 6 to 8 weeks.[52] Severe cases can be managed with erythrocytapheresis.[62]

Transfusion practices must be altered in the time surrounding an ABO-mismatched HSCT. Red blood cells and products containing plasma should be compatible with both donor and recipient cells.[52] For example, a type B recipient receiving a type A HSCT would be transfused only with type O red blood cells and type AB plasma. Once the individual's blood type has switched completely to the recipient type and antibodies are undetectable, transfusions may be performed as appropriate for the new blood type.[52]

Solid Organ Transplant

Because ABH molecules are expressed ubiquitously on endothelial cells, transplant of an ABO-incompatible organ can result in hyperacute rejection. However, advances in management have made it possible to transplant ABO-incompatible organs.[63] Major incompatible ABO liver transplants can be successful in both children and adults.[64] Because ABH expression and immune responses are lower in young pediatric patients, major incompatible ABO heart transplants can be performed in infants.[65]

Protocols for ABO-incompatible organ transplant involve depleting recipient antibodies with plasmapheresis followed by a variety of immunosuppressive regimens.[66–68] ABO incompatibility may result in slightly higher rates of graft loss; but with new protocols, there is no difference in survival.[69]

Passenger lymphocyte syndrome occurs in solid organ transplant when B lymphocytes are implanted with the graft.[70] Treatment of passenger lymphocyte syndrome is the same as for HSCT.

Intravenous Immunoglobulin

Because intravenous (IV) immunoglobulin is derived from plasma, isohemagglutinins are part of the immunoglobulin preparation. In the minor incompatible setting (non–group O), these infusions cause significant hemolysis in 1% of recipients.[71]

CLINICAL MANAGEMENT
Symptoms

The most common presentations of ABO-incompatible hemolysis are fever, chills, back pain, skin flushing, and hematuria, although other symptoms may occur (**Box 2**).[40] In the setting of blood transfusion, symptoms vary depending on total volume transfused: receiving more than 50 mL is associated with more severe reactions, including death.[72]

Box 2
Clinical findings in ABO-incompatible transfusion reactions

- Fever/chills
- Back pain
- Agitation/apprehension
- Dyspnea
- Tachycardia
- Oliguria
- Hypotension
- Hypertension
- Renal failure
- Diffuse intravascular coagulation
- Seizures

Treatment

If a hemolytic transfusion reaction is suspected, the transfusion must be stopped immediately and IV access should be maintained with 0.9% saline. An identity check of both the patient and the blood product should be performed at the bedside, and the blood product should be returned to the blood bank for a laboratory evaluation.[73] Immediate laboratory testing includes complete blood count (CBC), direct antiglobulin test, serum bilirubin, haptoglobin, lactate dehydrogenase, and urine hemoglobin (**Table 1**).[73,74]

Supportive treatment (**Box 3**) is derived in part from literature on rhabdomyolysis management[75] and involves management of diffuse intravascular coagulation and prevention of kidney failure. Aggressive hydration with IV crystalloid is recommended to prevent renal failure.[76] The addition of bicarbonate to IV fluids is recommended to counteract acidosis and to alkalinize the urine for hemoglobin solubilization.[77] The utility of diuresis with mannitol or loop diuretics to maintain kidney function is not clear.[76–78]

Prevention

For red blood cell transfusion, prevention of ABO incompatibility is paramount. Many cases with errors have problems at multiple steps, often involving incorrect patient identification. Mislabeled patient specimens result in a 40-fold increase in blood typing discrepancies,[79] which is why blood banks refuse any specimen that is not perfectly labeled.[80]

Table 1
Laboratory findings in the setting of ABO incompatibility

Laboratory Test	Changes Observed in Hemolytic Anemia
CBC	Decreased hematocrit Increased reticulocyte count (subacute)
Serum bilirubin	Increased bilirubin, primarily indirect
Serum haptoglobin	Decreased
Serum lactate dehydrogenase	Elevated
Urine hemoglobin	Present
Direct antiglobulin test	Positive

> **Box 3**
> **Treatment of ABO-incompatible hemolytic transfusion reactions**
>
> - Discontinue transfusion
> - Hydrate with IV fluids
> - Initiate laboratory workup
> - Consider plasma and platelet repletion in disseminated intravascular coagulation
> - Consider diuresis and/or urine alkalinization

Within the blood bank, incorrect blood labeling or unit selection is a cause of errors.[72] To decrease the rate of clerical errors, modern blood products include a large label describing the ABO group of the product (**Fig. 7**).

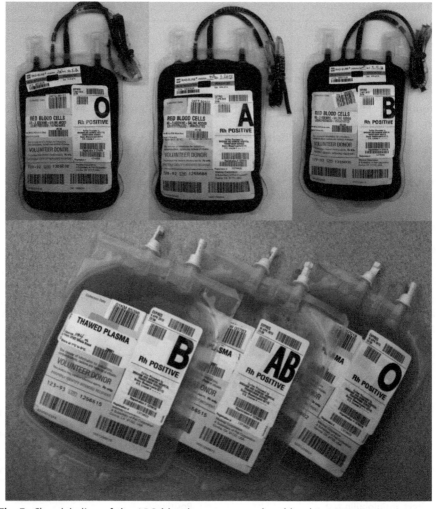

Fig. 7. Clear labeling of the ABO blood group on modern blood groups.

The bedside check is the last opportunity to prevent a serious error by verifying that the blood product is issued to the correct patient. However, in one study, rigorous verification of identification at the bedside occurred in only one-quarter of cases.[81] Several interventions have been attempted to increase verification, such as scanning a bar code at the bedside to ensure a final verification of identity.[82–84]

SUMMARY

Transfusion of blood products can be lifesaving; but appropriate ABO matching is crucial to prevent life-threatening hemolytic reactions, which are largely driven by complement activation. With systems in place to ensure that the blood product is matched to the recipient, ABO-incompatible hemolytic reactions are rare. There are additional clinical settings for ABO incompatibility that are unavoidable but manageable. Prevention and supportive treatment of ABO-incompatible hemolysis is necessary to ensure patient safety.

REFERENCES

1. Denis J. An extract of a letter of J. Denis Prof. of philosophy and mathematics April 2. 1667. Philosophical Trans 1666;2:617–23.
2. Blundell J. Experiments on the transfusion of blood by the syringe. Med Chir Trans 1818;9(Pt 1):56–92.
3. Walter WA. Successful case of transfusion of blood after severe post partum haemorrhage. Br Med J 1882;2(1131):415.
4. Soden JA. Case of haemorrhage from inversion of the uterus in which the operation of transfusion was successfully performed, with remarks on the employment of transfusion generally. Med Chir Trans 1852;35:413–35.
5. Schwarz HP, Dorner F. Karl Landsteiner and his major contributions to haematology. Br J Haematol 2003;121(4):556–65.
6. Hess JR, Schmidt PJ. The first blood banker: Oswald Hope Robertson. Transfusion 2000;40(1):110–3.
7. Thalhimer W, Tisdall LH. A review of the blood donor service of the American Red Cross. Am J Surg 1946;72:300–6.
8. Bianco T, Farmer BJ, Sage RE, et al. Loss of red cell A, B, and H antigens is frequent in myeloid malignancies. Blood 2001;97(11):3633–9.
9. Judd WJ, Annesley TM. The acquired-B phenomenon. Transfus Med Rev 1996; 10(2):111–7.
10. Garratty G. Blood groups and disease: a historical perspective. Transfus Med Rev 2000;14(4):291–301.
11. Ravn V, Dabelsteen E. Tissue distribution of histo-blood group antigens. APMIS 2000;108(1):1–28.
12. Daniels G. Human blood groups: Geoff Daniels; foreword by Ruth Sanger. 3rd edition. Chichester (United Kingdom), West Sussex (United Kingdom): John Wiley & Sons; 2013.
13. Le Pendu J, Cartron JP, Lemieux RU, et al. The presence of at least two different H-blood-group-related beta-D-gal alpha-2-L-fucosyltransferases in human serum and the genetics of blood group H substances. Am J Hum Genet 1985; 37(4):749–60.
14. Larsen RD, Ernst LK, Nair RP, et al. Molecular cloning, sequence, and expression of a human GDP-L-fucose:beta-D-galactoside 2-alpha-L-fucosyltransferase cDNA that can form the H blood group antigen. Proc Natl Acad Sci U S A 1990;87(17):6674–8.

15. Rege WP, Painter TJ, Watkins WM, et al. Isolation of serologically active fucose-containing oligosaccharides from human blood-group H substance. Nature 1964; 203:360–3.
16. Yunis EJ, Svardal JM, Bridges RA. Genetics of the Bombay phenotype. Blood 1969;33(1):124–32.
17. Yamamoto F, Clausen H, White T, et al. Molecular genetic basis of the histo-blood group ABO system. Nature 1990;345(6272):229–33.
18. Clausen H, Bennett EP, Grunnet N. Molecular genetics of ABO histo-blood groups. Transfus Clin Biol 1994;1(2):79–89.
19. Watkins WM, Greenwell P, Yates AD, et al. Regulation of expression of carbohydrate blood group antigens. Biochimie 1988;70(11):1597–611.
20. Reid ME, Lomas-Francis C, Olsson ML. The blood group antigen facts book. 3rd edition. Boston: Elsevier/Academic Press; 2012.
21. Preece AF, Strahan KM, Devitt J, et al. Expression of ABO or related antigenic carbohydrates on viral envelopes leads to neutralization in the presence of serum containing specific natural antibodies and complement. Blood 2002;99(7):2477–82.
22. Avrameas S, Selmi C. Natural autoantibodies in the physiology and pathophysiology of the immune system. J Autoimmun 2013;41:46–9.
23. Mannoor K, Xu Y, Chen C. Natural autoantibodies and associated B cells in immunity and autoimmunity. Autoimmunity 2013;46(2):138–47.
24. Obukhova P, Korchagina E, Henry S, et al. Natural anti-A and anti-B of the ABO system: allo- and autoantibodies have different epitope specificity. Transfusion 2012;52(4):860–9.
25. Rieben R, Tucci A, Nydegger UE, et al. Self tolerance to human A and B histo-blood group antigens exists at the B cell level and cannot be broken by potent polyclonal B cell activation in vitro. Eur J Immunol 1992;22(10):2713–7.
26. Spalter SH, Kaveri SV, Bonnin E, et al. Normal human serum contains natural antibodies reactive with autologous ABO blood group antigens. Blood 1999; 93(12):4418–24.
27. Stussi G, Huggel K, Lutz HU, et al. Isotype-specific detection of ABO blood group antibodies using a novel flow cytometric method. Br J Haematol 2005;130(6): 954–63.
28. Reeves PR, Hobbs M, Valvano MA, et al. Bacterial polysaccharide synthesis and gene nomenclature. Trends Microbiol 1996;4(12):495–503.
29. Springer GF, Williamson P, Brandes WC. Blood group activity of gram-negative bacteria. J Exp Med 1961;113(6):1077–93.
30. Hansson J, Bosco N, Favre L, et al. Influence of gut microbiota on mouse B2 B cell ontogeny and function. Mol Immunol 2010;48(9–10):1091–101.
31. Springer GF, Horton RE, Forbes M. Origin of anti-human blood group B agglutinins in white leghorn chicks. J Exp Med 1959;110(2):221–44 [in Undetermined Language].
32. Springer GF, Horton RE. Blood group isoantibody stimulation in man by feeding blood group-active bacteria. J Clin Invest 1969;48(7):1280–91.
33. Daniel-Johnson J, Leitman S, Klein H, et al. Probiotic-associated high-titer anti-B in a group A platelet donor as a cause of severe hemolytic transfusion reactions. Transfusion 2009;49(9):1845–9.
34. Miler JJ, Novotny P, Walker PD, et al. Neisseria gonorrhoeae and ABO isohemagglutinins. Infect Immun 1977;15(3):713–9.
35. Atkinson JP, Frank MM. Studies on the in vivo effects of antibody. Interaction of IgM antibody and complement in the immune clearance and destruction of erythrocytes in man. J Clin Invest 1974;54(2):339–48.

36. Kurlander RJ, Rosse WF, Logue GL. Quantitative influence of antibody and complement coating of red cells on monocyte-mediated cell lysis. J Clin Invest 1978;61(5):1309–19.
37. Lucisano Valim YM, Lachmann PJ. The effect of antibody isotype and antigenic epitope density on the complement-fixing activity of immune complexes: a systematic study using chimaeric anti-NIP antibodies with human Fc regions. Clin Exp Immunol 1991;84(1):1–8.
38. Markiewski MM, Nilsson B, Ekdahl KN, et al. Complement and coagulation: strangers or partners in crime? Trends Immunol 2007;28(4):184–92.
39. Rother RP, Bell L, Hillmen P, et al. The clinical sequelae of intravascular hemolysis and extracellular plasma hemoglobin: a novel mechanism of human disease. JAMA 2005;293(13):1653–62.
40. Sazama K. Reports of 355 transfusion-associated deaths: 1976 through 1985. Transfusion 1990;30(7):583–90.
41. Stainsby D, Russell J, Cohen H, et al. Reducing adverse events in blood transfusion. Br J Haematol 2005;131(1):8–12.
42. Linden JV, Wagner K, Voytovich AE, et al. Transfusion errors in New York State: an analysis of 10 years' experience. Transfusion 2000;40(10):1207–13.
43. Levine P. The protective action of ABO incompatibility on Rh isoimmunization and Rh hemolytic disease-theoretical and clinical implications. Am J Hum Genet 1959;11(2 Pt 2):418.
44. Donohue WL, Wake EJ. Effect of abo incompatibility on pregnancy-induced Rh isoimmunization. Can Med Assoc J 1964;90:1–5.
45. Roberts IA. The changing face of haemolytic disease of the newborn. Early Hum Dev 2008;84(8):515–23.
46. Bakkeheim E, Bergerud U, Schmidt-Melbye AC, et al. Maternal IgG anti-A and anti-B titres predict outcome in ABO-incompatibility in the neonate. Acta Paediatr 2009;98(12):1896–901.
47. Triulzi DJ, Assmann SF, Strauss RG, et al. The impact of platelet transfusion characteristics on posttransfusion platelet increments and clinical bleeding in patients with hypoproliferative thrombocytopenia. Blood 2012;119(23):5553–62.
48. Pavenski K, Warkentin TE, Shen H, et al. Posttransfusion platelet count increments after ABO-compatible versus ABO-incompatible platelet transfusions in noncancer patients: an observational study. Transfusion 2010;50(7):1552–60.
49. Fung MK, Downes KA, Shulman IA. Transfusion of platelets containing ABO-incompatible plasma: a survey of 3156 North American laboratories. Arch Pathol Lab Med 2007;131(6):909–16.
50. Dunbar NM, Ornstein DL, Dumont LJ. ABO incompatible platelets: risks versus benefit. Curr Opin Hematol 2012;19(6):475–9.
51. Karafin MS, Blagg L, Tobian AA, et al. ABO antibody titers are not predictive of hemolytic reactions due to plasma-incompatible platelet transfusions. Transfusion 2012;52(10):2087–93.
52. Booth GS, Gehrie EA, Bolan CD, et al. Clinical guide to ABO-incompatible allogeneic stem cell transplantation. Biol Blood Marrow Transplant 2013;19(8):1152–8.
53. Seebach JD, Stussi G, Passweg JR, et al. ABO blood group barrier in allogeneic bone marrow transplantation revisited. Biol Blood Marrow Transplant 2005;11(12):1006–13.
54. Kollman C, Howe CW, Anasetti C, et al. Donor characteristics as risk factors in recipients after transplantation of bone marrow from unrelated donors: the effect of donor age. Blood 2001;98(7):2043–51.

55. Kimura F, Sato K, Kobayashi S, et al. Impact of ABO-blood group incompatibility on the outcome of recipients of bone marrow transplants from unrelated donors in the Japan marrow donor program. Haematologica 2008;93(11):1686–93.

56. Michallet M, Le QH, Mohty M, et al. Predictive factors for outcomes after reduced intensity conditioning hematopoietic stem cell transplantation for hematological malignancies: a 10-year retrospective analysis from the Societe Francaise de Greffe de Moelle et de Therapie Cellulaire. Exp Hematol 2008; 36(5):535–44.

57. Blacklock HA, Katz F, Michalevicz R, et al. A and B blood group antigen expression on mixed colony cells and erythroid precursors: relevance for human allogeneic bone marrow transplantation. Br J Haematol 1984;58(2):267–76.

58. Rowley SD. Hematopoietic stem cell transplantation between red cell incompatible donor-recipient pairs. Bone Marrow Transplant 2001;28(4):315–21.

59. Curley C, Pillai E, Mudie K, et al. Outcomes after major or bidirectional ABO-mismatched allogeneic hematopoietic progenitor cell transplantation after pretransplant isoagglutinin reduction with donor-type secretor plasma with or without plasma exchange. Transfusion 2012;52(2):291–7.

60. Gmur JP, Burger J, Schaffner A, et al. Pure red cell aplasia of long duration complicating major ABO-incompatible bone marrow transplantation. Blood 1990;75(1):290–5.

61. Hows J, Beddow K, Gordon-Smith E, et al. Donor-derived red blood cell antibodies and immune hemolysis after allogeneic bone marrow transplantation. Blood 1986;67(1):177–81.

62. Worel N, Greinix HT, Supper V, et al. Prophylactic red blood cell exchange for prevention of severe immune hemolysis in minor ABO-mismatched allogeneic peripheral blood progenitor cell transplantation after reduced-intensity conditioning. Transfusion 2007;47(8):1494–502.

63. Magee CC. Transplantation across previously incompatible immunological barriers. Transpl Int 2006;19(2):87–97.

64. Raut V, Uemoto S. Management of ABO-incompatible living-donor liver transplantation: past and present trends. Surg Today 2011;41(3):317–22.

65. Urschel S, Larsen IM, Kirk R, et al. ABO-incompatible heart transplantation in early childhood: an international multicenter study of clinical experiences and limits. J Heart Lung Transplant 2013;32(3):285–92.

66. Takahashi K, Saito K, Takahara S, et al. Excellent long-term outcome of ABO-incompatible living donor kidney transplantation in Japan. Am J Transplant 2004;4(7):1089–96.

67. Sonnenday CJ, Warren DS, Cooper M, et al. Plasmapheresis, CMV hyperimmune globulin, and anti-CD20 allow ABO-incompatible renal transplantation without splenectomy. Am J Transplant 2004;4(8):1315–22.

68. Tyden G, Kumlien G, Genberg H, et al. ABO incompatible kidney transplantations without splenectomy, using antigen-specific immunoadsorption and rituximab. Am J Transplant 2005;5(1):145–8.

69. Montgomery JR, Berger JC, Warren DS, et al. Outcomes of ABO-incompatible kidney transplantation in the United States. Transplantation 2012;93(6):603–9.

70. Nadarajah L, Ashman N, Thuraisingham R, et al. Literature review of passenger lymphocyte syndrome following renal transplantation and two case reports. Am J Transplant 2013;13(6):1594–600.

71. Daw Z, Padmore R, Neurath D, et al. Hemolytic transfusion reactions after administration of intravenous immune (gamma) globulin: a case series analysis. Transfusion 2008;48(8):1598–601.

72. Janatpour KA, Kalmin ND, Jensen HM, et al. Clinical outcomes of ABO-incompatible RBC transfusions. Am J Clin Pathol 2008;129(2):276–81.
73. Strobel E. Hemolytic transfusion reactions. Transfus Med Hemother 2008;35(5): 346–53.
74. Petz LD, Garratty G, Petz LD. Immune hemolytic anemias. 2nd edition. Philadelphia: Churchill Livingstone; 2004.
75. Zimmerman JL, Shen MC. Rhabdomyolysis. Chest 2013;144(3):1058–65.
76. Lameire N, Van Biesen W, Vanholder R. Acute renal failure. Lancet 2005; 365(9457):417–30.
77. Bosch X, Poch E, Grau JM. Rhabdomyolysis and acute kidney injury. N Engl J Med 2009;361(1):62–72.
78. Kellum JA. The use of diuretics and dopamine in acute renal failure: a systematic review of the evidence. Crit Care 1997;1(2):53–9.
79. Lumadue JA, Boyd JS, Ness PM. Adherence to a strict specimen-labeling policy decreases the incidence of erroneous blood grouping of blood bank specimens. Transfusion 1997;37(11–12):1169–72.
80. Dzik WH. New technology for transfusion safety. Br J Haematol 2007;136(2): 181–90.
81. Novis DA, Miller KA, Howanitz PJ, et al. Audit of transfusion procedures in 660 hospitals. A College of American Pathologists Q-Probes study of patient identification and vital sign monitoring frequencies in 16494 transfusions. Arch Pathol Lab Med 2003;127(5):541–8.
82. Porcella A, Walker K. Patient safety with blood products administration using wireless and bar-code technology. AMIA Annu Symp Proc 2005;614–8.
83. Murphy MF, Casbard AC, Ballard S, et al. Prevention of bedside errors in transfusion medicine (PROBE-TM) study: a cluster-randomized, matched-paired clinical areas trial of a simple intervention to reduce errors in the pretransfusion bedside check. Transfusion 2007;47(5):771–80.
84. Murphy MF, Kay JD. Bar code identification for transfusion safety. Curr Opin Hematol 2004;11(5):334–8.

Warm Autoimmune Hemolytic Anemia

Rakhi Naik, MD, MHS

KEYWORDS

- Autoimmune hemolytic anemia • Spherocyte • Direct antiglobulin test
- Complement

KEY POINTS

- Warm autoimmune hemolytic anemia (AIHA) is a rare disease, occurring in both idiopathic and secondary forms; common secondary etiologies include lymphoproliferative disorders, autoimmune disease, and drugs.
- Diagnosis involves the presence of markers of hemolysis and a positive direct Coombs test, which most commonly reveals red blood cell–bound immunoglobulin G antibodies with or without C3 complement.
- Erythrocyte destruction in warm AIHA is mediated by extravascular phagocytosis in the spleen and, in some cases, may involve complement-mediated mechanisms.
- Complement may exacerbate intravascular and extravascular hemolysis and is often a major contributor to severe forms of warm hemolytic crisis.
- First-line therapy includes corticosteroids followed by splenectomy or rituximab. The role of anticomplement agents in warm AIHA is unknown.

INTRODUCTION

Autoimmune hemolytic anemia (AIHA) is defined as the destruction of circulating red blood cells (RBCs) in the setting of anti-RBC autoantibodies.[1] The *in vivo* and *in vitro* behavior of these autoantibodies allows for classification of AIHA into 3 forms: a warm type that causes agglutination of the blood at 37°C, a cold agglutinin that optimally reacts at 0°C to 5°C, and mixed-type disease that displays features of both.[2] Warm AIHA is often suspected in the patient who develops hemolytic anemia with characteristic morphologic findings of microspherocytes on the peripheral smear. The disease occurs in both idiopathic and secondary settings, making investigation of potential underlying etiologies essential. The diagnosis ultimately requires confirmation with identification of an anti-RBC autoantibody by direct antiglobulin tests

The author has nothing to disclose.
Division of Hematology, Department of Medicine, The Johns Hopkins University School of Medicine, 1830 East Monument Street, Baltimore, MD 21230, USA
E-mail address: rakhi@jhmi.edu

Hematol Oncol Clin N Am 29 (2015) 445–453
http://dx.doi.org/10.1016/j.hoc.2015.01.001
0889-8588/15/$ – see front matter © 2015 Elsevier Inc. All rights reserved.

(DAT) and by the presence or absence of complement fractions, which also contribute to the pathogenesis of disease.[2,3] Warm AIHA is most often associated with a positive DAT for RBC-bound immunoglobulin (Ig)G and/or C3.[2,4]

History

The first cases of acquired warm hemolytic anemia were identified in the 1890s by Georges Hayem, who described a series of patients with the hallmark features of chronic jaundice, anemia, and splenomegaly.[5] He noted that the type of jaundice was marked by a lack of biliary pigment, differentiating the condition from usual hepatic etiologies. However, despite the early initial recognition of the clinical presentation, the syndrome was not widely recognized until the mid-20th century.[5] In 1940, Dameshek and Schwartz compiled previously published cases of acquired hemolytic jaundice, leading to the hypothesis that the disease was secondary to direct RBC lysis and that the severity of disease was related to the degree of hemolysis.[5,6] Around the same time, interest in RBC immunobiology began to peak, and by 1945, the antiglobulin test was developed by an astute veterinarian, Robin Coombs. This essential blood-banking test was first used to identify pathogenic RBC antibodies in cases of hemolytic disease of the newborn,[5,7] and both the direct and indirect antiglobulin tests now bear his name. The role of nonimmunoglobulin elements, such as complement, in the pathobiology of disease was not recognized until the 1950s.[5]

Epidemiology

AIHA is known to be a rare disorder, although the non–disease-specific prevalence and incidence rates have not been widely reported. The incidence seems to be low at 0.8 to 3 cases per 100,000 person-years,[4,8,9] resulting in an overall prevalence of about 17 cases per 100,000 individuals.[10] Warm-reacting autoantibodies comprise the majority of cases of AIHA.[11] Among cases of warm AIHA, primary or idiopathic disease occurs in about 50% of cases,[4] with the remainder occurring in the setting of an underlying malignant, autoimmune, infectious, or drug triggers. For idiopathic warm AIHA, females are more commonly affected than males and are generally affected in their fourth or fifth decade.[4] The demographic prevalence of secondary causes varies widely and is primarily driven by the underlying disease.

DIAGNOSIS
Clinical Symptoms

AIHA is a clinicopathologic diagnosis that requires the presence of clinical features of hemolysis as well as serologic positivity for RBC-directed antibodies and/or complement fractions. The clinical spectrum of disease in warm AIHA is wide, with some patients presenting with mild, asymptomatic anemia and others presenting with a life-threatening hemolytic crisis. Common features include symptoms related to the degree of anemia, such as fatigue, weakness, pallor, and dyspnea on exertion, and symptoms related to hemolysis, such as jaundice, hemoglobinuria, or splenic fullness.

Laboratory Evaluation

Serologic diagnosis of warm AIHA requires confirmation of hemolytic anemia and pathologic anti-RBC immunoglobulins with or without RBC-bound complement. The hemolysis associated with warm AIHA is classically extravascular, or occurring in the spleen, although intravascular hemolysis is also common and may account for many of the fulminant cases of warm AIHA.[4] Near universal laboratory features of hemolysis include low hemoglobin, elevated reticulocyte count, and elevated lactate dehydrogenase levels. Depleted haptoglobin levels and elevated indirect bilirubin may also been seen in a majority of cases.[12] The anemia may often be macrocytic because of the degree of reticulocytosis.[8] In a series of 69 cases of primary and secondary warm AIHA, the mean hematocrit at presentation was 25% with a mean reticulocyte percentage of 14% to 18%.[13] The peripheral smear often demonstrates microspherocytes, which are thought to be a manifestation of the reduced surface-to-volume ratio caused by phagocytosis of immunoglobulin-coated RBCs in the spleen (**Fig. 1**).[14] Howell-Jolly bodies also may be seen after splenectomy.

The primary laboratory method for the diagnosis of AIHA is the direct antiglobulin (Coombs) test (DAT). The DAT is performed by adding a poly-specific antiglobulin reagent to a washed, suspended sample of the patient's blood.[1] Agglutination of the cells after centrifugation confirms that the antiglobulin has resulted in crosslinking of antibody-coated RBCs.[1,4] A similar method is used for the detection of C3d-coated RBCs. An indirect antiglobulin test can also be used to detect unbound antibodies in the RBC eluate. In the indirect method, the serum and/or RBC eluate are incubated with donor RBCs. Agglutination after addition of antiglobulin suggests that circulating RBC-specific immunoglobulins in the patient's serum have bound to the donor RBCs.[1] This method can be used to differentiate autoantibodies from alloantibodies because autoantibodies tend to be panagglutinins (ie, they react with all panel RBCs), whereas alloantibodies are RBC antigen specific.[4] The most common DAT findings in warm AIHA are +IgG (and rarely IgA or IgM) with or without +C3. The serum and indirect DAT findings will reveal a panagglutinating IgG.[2,4]

Although positive DAT findings are suggestive of AIHA, the presence of serologic markers of AIHA in the absence of clinical hemolysis can occur in many settings. Approximately 0.1% of healthy blood donors and up to 8% of asymptomatic hospitalized patients may have a positive DAT.[4,15,16] A positive DAT also occurs frequently in the setting of delayed transfusion reactions and after administration of intravenous immunoglobulin (IVIG).[17,18] In contrast, a false-negative DAT is rare, but may occur in a small proportion (3%) of patients with AIHA, possibly secondary to low titer immunoglobulins, low-affinity autoantibodies, or the presence of warm IgA or IgM antibodies.[19] In these cases, warm AIHA should be suspected if the smear demonstrates microspherocytes, the clinical presentation is typical of warm AIHA, or if the patient responds to empiric immunosuppressive therapy. Additional testing may detect the culprit autoantibody in DAT-negative AIHA; for example, IgA-specific

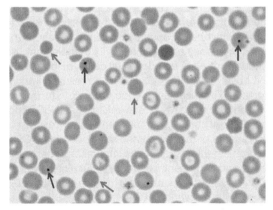

Fig. 1. Microphotograph of a peripheral smear in a patient with warm autoimmune hemolytic anemia status post splenectomy, showing prominent microspherocytes (*blue arrows*) and Howell-Jolly bodies (*red arrows*).

antiglobulin can be used to diagnose IgA-mediated disease and high sensitivity assays, such as microcolumn DAT techniques or flow cytometry can be used to detect low-titer or low-affinity disease.[20]

Although IVIG administration may lead to Coombs positivity in the absence of hemolysis, clinically significant reactions, including severe intravascular hemolysis, have been reported. These reactions are thought to occur in the setting of passive transfer of major and minor blood group antibodies, such that those with non-O blood groups are more susceptible to hemolytic reactions.[21] Because each batch of IVIG contains different immunoglobulins, it is not easy to predict the risk of developing clinical hemolysis. Suggested approaches include cross-matching before IVIG infusion or monitoring laboratory parameters, including DAT and hemolysis serologies after infusion, so that further treatment can be withheld if signs of hemolysis are present.[21]

ETIOLOGY
Autoantibody Response

The pathophysiology of autoantibody generation in AIHA is poorly understood but likely involves the interplay of multiple complex processes, including immune dysregulation and abnormal autoantigen response.[3] The most common target for warm agglutinins are Rhesus (Rh) polypeptides on the RBC surface,[22] and despite their association with clonal lymphoproliferative disorders, these warm autoantibodies are usually polyclonal.[4] The underlying stimulus for autoantibody production in AIHA may involve molecular mimicry secondary to cross-reactivity of endogenous RBC and environmental antigens.[3,22] Alternatively, abnormal processing of autoantigens in the setting of environmental factors may overcome self-tolerance.[23] Immune dysfunction of B and T cells also likely contributes to autoimmunity in AIHA, because immunodeficiency states such infection with human immunodeficiency virus and lymphoproliferative neoplasms such as chronic lymphocytic leukemia (CLL), are often associated with warm AIHA and DAT positivity.[24,25]

The mechanism of RBC destruction in the setting of warm autoantibodies involves the recognition of the Fc portion of the IgG molecule by tissue macrophages in the spleen.[4] The degree of extravascular hemolysis depends the antibody titer, IgG subclass, and presence of bound complement, which can also be recognized and cleared by the spleen.[26]

Role of Complement

Unlike in cold agglutinins disease, which is mediated exclusively by IgM, warm AIHA is only variably associated with directly bound complement because the most commonly involved autoantibody, IgG, does not universally fix complement. Nonetheless, many cases of IgG-mediated warm AIHA and nearly all cases of IgM-mediated warm agglutinins demonstrate a positive DAT for C3, which can result in intravascular hemolysis and potentiate ongoing extravascular phagocytosis.[26,27] In IgG-mediated disease, the subclass of the pathologic antibody is relevant; IgG1 and IgG3 subclasses are associated with an increased ability to bind complement.[21] Intravascular hemolysis is mediated by the cytotoxic effects of the membrane attack complex (C5b-C9), which is the end product of the complement cascade. The intravascular hemolysis related to complement can be robust and is present frequently in fulminant cases of warm AIHA. In fact, mortality rates in IgM-related warm autoimmune disease are high, likely owing to the degree of complement activation.[28] Serum- and RBC-bound complement regulatory proteins, however, may mitigate the degree of intravascular hemolysis in many cases of warm AIHA, because C3 DAT positivity is often detected without evidence of intravascular RBC lysis.[1]

ASSOCIATED CONDITIONS

Secondary causes of warm AIHA are diverse and include malignant, autoimmune, infectious/immunodeficiency, and drug causes (**Table 1**). Of the secondary triggers for warm AIHA, lymphoproliferative disorders are among the most common and include CLL, non-Hodgkin lymphomas, and myelomas. Like many paraneoplastic syndromes, the presence of AIHA may precede the development of a clinically apparent malignancy.[29] The most frequently associated hematologic malignancy with warm AIHA is CLL, with approximately 4% to 10% of CLL cases being complicated by hemolytic disease.[30,31] Treatment with purine analogs such as fludarabine may exacerbate or trigger severe hemolytic reactions in patients with CLL.[32] DAT positivity in the absence of clinically relevant hemolysis may also occur in up to 35% of patients in the setting of known malignant disease.[31]

Autoimmune disease, especially systemic lupus erythematosus, is also associated commonly with warm AIHA, occurring in up to one-third of patients in some series.[33] In fact, warm AIHA is included in the criteria for a diagnosis of systemic lupus erythematosus.[34] Immune dysregulatory states such as human immunodeficiency virus and common variable immunodeficiency may result in a paradoxical increase in hematologic autoimmunity including warm AIHA, despite an underlying decreased responsiveness to infection.[24,35]

Medications may also trigger warm AIHA in a drug-dependent manner. In drug-related cases, medication cessation usually alleviates the hemolysis. The mechanism of autoimmune destruction in drug-induced warm AIHA includes the binding of autoantibodies to RBCs only in the presence of drug (hapten mechanism) or the deposition and activation of complement on the RBC surface in the presence of drug alone (ternary complex mechanism).[1,36] These complement-inducing drug reactions often lead to fulminant intravascular hemolysis. Rarely, non–drug-dependent RBC autoantibody production can be triggered by the introduction of a medication, but even in these cases, drug cessation is effective in stopping the hemolytic reaction.[1]

Warm AIHA directed against recipient RBCs may also occur in the setting of allogeneic stem cell transplantation and solid organ transplantation owing to passenger lymphocyte syndrome.[8] This condition is thought to occur secondary to RBC-directed autoantibody production against recipient cells generated by primed B lymphocytes in the donor tissue. Clinically severe hemolysis usually occurs within the first 2 weeks after transplantation in the setting of major ABO incompatibility, but may be observed with minor antigen incompatibility as well.[37]

Table 1
Common secondary causes of warm autoimmune hemolytic anemia

Category	Condition
Malignancy	Chronic lymphocytic leukemia
	Hodgkin/non-Hodgkin lymphoma
	Multiple myeloma
	Solid tumors (ovarian)
Autoimmune disease	Systemic lupus erythematosus
	Ulcerative colitis
Immunodeficiency states	Human immunodeficiency virus
	Common variable immune deficiency
Other	Drugs
	Posthematopoietic or solid organ transplant

TREATMENT
Transfusion

The first determination for patients who present with AIHA is the need for transfusion. Because the autoantibodies in warm AIHA often cause panagglutination of donor RBCs, true cross-matching is usually not possible. However, transfusion can often be safely administered with ABO and Rh-D matched blood in urgent cases.[8] Fulminant hemolytic crisis, which usually occurs in cases with robust complement-mediated intravascular hemolysis, such as IgM-mediated warm AIHA, can result in significant morbidity and mortality.[28] Reticulocytopenia in the early phase of disease is common and can blunt erythrocyte recovery; therefore, transfusion should not be withheld, especially in the setting of severe anemia, hypoxia, or hemodynamic compromise.[38] Initial slow infusion is recommended to ensure that an acute transfusion reaction does not occur. Although much of the transfused blood may be hemolyzed owing to the panreactive autoantibodies, the transient increase in oxygen-carrying capacity can be essential.[1,8]

An approach to transfusion in a patient with warm AIHA includes[8]:

- Transfusion of best-matched or least incompatible blood.
  - Full cross-matching often not possible owing to panagglutinating properties of warm autoantibodies.
  - ABO– and Rh-D–matched units in those unlikely to have existing alloantibodies such as females without prior pregnancy and transfusion or males without a history of transfusion.
  - Extended phenotype matching for additional Rh subgroups (C, c, E, e, Kell, Kidd, S, s) in nonurgent cases or in cases where a high risk of alloimmunization is suspected.
- Test infusion of blood to monitor of acute transfusion reactions.
  - Initial infusion of 20 to 30 mL blood.
  - Observe for 20 to 30 minutes.
  - Continue with planned transfusion if no reaction.

First-Line Treatment

Pharmacologic treatment for warm AIHA is based mostly on expert opinion; formal trials are lacking. As per general consensus, steroids at a dose of 1 mg/kg per day of prednisone should be used as first-line treatment, with nearly 80% of patients achieving a response with corticosteroids alone.[2,8,39] The goal of therapy is to increase baseline hemoglobin levels to 9 to 10 g/dL, which is usually achieved within the first 3 weeks of treatment. A slow taper over several months is often required to avoid symptomatic relapse. Although response rates to steroid are high, most adults require long-term steroid therapy to maintain remission, with up to 20% requiring doses of more than 15 mg/d.[8] The mechanism of steroid efficacy in warm AIHA is not only owing to a decrease in antibody production, but may also relate to its suppressive effects on tissue macrophage phagocytosis and direct effect on autoantibody RBC affinity.[2]

Second-Line Treatment

For patients who do not respond to steroids, require high long-term doses, or have unacceptable side effects, second-line therapy is required. The 2 most accepted second-line therapies for warm AIHA include splenectomy and rituximab therapy. Splenectomy demonstrates success rates of approximately 50%, although sustained low-dose steroids may also be required to maintain a durable remission.[40,41]

Continued compensated intravascular or extravascular hemolysis after splenectomy is not uncommon.[1] Although the risk of infectious complications can be mitigated by vaccination, thrombotic complications can occur in up to one-quarter of splenectomized patients with AIHA.[40]

A therapeutic alternative to splenectomy for second-line therapy is rituximab, a monoclonal against antibody CD20 on B cells. Treatment regimens include standard dosing of 4 weekly infusions at 375 mg/m^2, autoimmune disease dosing of two times 1000 mg given 2 weeks apart, or even low fixed dose of 100 mg weekly for 4 doses.[12,20] Initial responses are observed in a majority (80%) of patients, but relapse in 1 to 3 years is common and may necessitate repeat therapy.[8,12] Rituximab has also been studied as first-line therapy with concurrent corticosteroid treatment and seems to induce more durable response than first-line treatment with corticosteroids alone.[42]

Other Therapies, Including Complement-Targeting Drugs

Literature on additional therapies for warm AIHA is scant. Treatment options in refractory cases include azathioprine or cyclophosphamide and other immunosuppressive drugs such as cyclosporine or mycophenolate mofetil; however, published case series on these regimens are small.[1,8] High-dose cyclophosphamide has been successful in severely refractory disease.[43] Complement-targeting agents have not yet been studied in warm AIHA, although effective use of a C1-esterase inhibitor and the terminal complement inhibitor, eculizumab, in warm IgM-mediated disease have been reported.[44,45] The utility in warm AIHA may extend beyond IgM disease, because it seems that anticomplement agents not only have activity against complement generation, but may have antiphagocytic activity as well.[46]

SUMMARY/DISCUSSION

Warm AIHA is an uncommon disorder caused by RBC-directed autoantibodies. RBC-bound complement, when present, may potentiate hemolysis and often presents with fulminant disease. Therapies are aimed generally at decreasing antibody production using immunosuppressive agents and reducing RBC phagocytosis in the spleen. The role for complement inhibitors in warm AIHA is not known currently.

REFERENCES

1. Packman CH. Hemolytic anemia due to warm autoantibodies. Blood Rev 2008; 22:17–31.
2. King KE, Ness PM. Treatment of autoimmune hemolytic anemia. Semin Hematol 2005;42:131–6.
3. Barros MM, Blajchman MA, Bordin JO. Warm autoimmune hemolytic anemia: recent progress in understanding the immunobiology and the treatment. Transfus Med Rev 2010;24:195–210.
4. Gehrs BC, Friedberg RC. Autoimmune hemolytic anemia. Am J Hematol 2002;69: 258–71.
5. Packman CH. The spherocytic haemolytic anaemias. Br J Haematol 2001;112: 888–99.
6. Dameshek W, Schwartz SO. Acute hemolytic anemia (acquired hemolytic icterus, acute type). Medicine 1940;19:231–327.
7. Coombs RR, Mourant AE, Race RR. A new test for the detection of weak and incomplete Rh agglutinins. Br J Exp Pathol 1945;26:255–66.
8. Lechner K, Jager U. How I treat autoimmune hemolytic anemias in adults. Blood 2010;116:1831–8.

9. Klein NP, Ray P, Carpenter D, et al. Rates of autoimmune diseases in Kaiser Permanente for use in vaccine adverse event safety studies. Vaccine 2010; 28:1062–8.

10. Eaton WW, Rose NR, Kalaydjian A, et al. Epidemiology of autoimmune diseases in Denmark. J Autoimmun 2007;29:1–9.

11. Sokol RJ, Hewitt S, Stamps BK. Autoimmune haemolysis: an 18-year study of 865 cases referred to a regional transfusion centre. Br Med J (Clin Res Ed) 1981;282: 2023–7.

12. Roumier M, Loustau V, Guillaud C, et al. Characteristics and outcome of warm autoimmune hemolytic anemia in adults: new insights based on a single-center experience with 60 patients. Am J Hematol 2014;89:E150–5.

13. Liesveld JL, Rowe JM, Lichtman MA. Variability of the erythropoietic response in autoimmune hemolytic anemia: analysis of 109 cases. Blood 1987;69:820–6.

14. Cartron JP, Agre P. Rh blood group antigens: protein and gene structure. Semin Hematol 1993;30:193–208.

15. Lau P, Haesler WE, Wurzel HA. Positive direct antiglobulin reaction in a patient population. Am J Clin Pathol 1976;65:368–75.

16. Judd WJ, Barnes BA, Steiner EA, et al. The evaluation of a positive direct antiglobulin test (autocontrol) in pretransfusion testing revisited. Transfusion 1986; 26:220–4.

17. Toy PT, Chin CA, Reid ME, et al. Factors associated with positive direct antiglobulin tests in pretransfusion patients: a case-control study. Vox Sang 1985;49: 215–20.

18. Clark JA, Tanley PC, Wallace CH. Evaluation of patients with positive direct antiglobulin tests and nonreactive eluates discovered during pretransfusion testing. Immunohematology 1992;8:9–12.

19. Sachs UJ, Roder L, Santoso S, et al. Does a negative direct antiglobulin test exclude warm autoimmune haemolytic anaemia? A prospective study of 504 cases. Br J Haematol 2006;132:655–6.

20. Zanella A, Barcellini W. Treatment of autoimmune hemolytic anemias. Haematologica 2014;99:1547–54.

21. Daw Z, Padmore R, Neurath D, et al. Hemolytic transfusion reactions after administration of intravenous immune (gamma) globulin: a case series analysis. Transfusion 2008;48:1598–601.

22. Barker RN, Hall AM, Standen GR, et al. Identification of T-cell epitopes on the Rhesus polypeptides in autoimmune hemolytic anemia. Blood 1997;90:2701–15.

23. Liu GY, Fairchild PJ, Smith RM, et al. Low avidity recognition of self-antigen by T cells permits escape from central tolerance. Immunity 1995;3:407–15.

24. De Angelis V, Biasinutto C, Pradella P, et al. Clinical significance of positive direct antiglobulin test in patients with HIV infection. Infection 1994;22:92–5.

25. Visco C, Barcellini W, Maura F, et al. Autoimmune cytopenias in chronic lymphocytic leukemia. Am J Hematol 2014;89:1055–62.

26. Ehlenberger AG, Nussenzweig V. The role of membrane receptors for C3b and C3d in phagocytosis. J Exp Med 1977;145:357–71.

27. Lay WH, Nussenzweig V. Receptors for complement of leukocytes. J Exp Med 1968;128:991–1009.

28. Arndt PA, Leger RM, Garratty G. Serologic findings in autoimmune hemolytic anemia associated with immunoglobulin M warm autoantibodies. Transfusion 2009; 49:235–42.

29. Fallah M, Liu X, Ji J, et al. Autoimmune diseases associated with non-Hodgkin lymphoma: a nationwide cohort study. Ann Oncol 2014;25:2025–30.

30. Mauro FR, Foa R, Cerretti R, et al. Autoimmune hemolytic anemia in chronic lymphocytic leukemia: clinical, therapeutic, and prognostic features. Blood 2000;95: 2786–92.
31. Ricci F, Tedeschi A, Vismara E, et al. Should a positive direct antiglobulin test be considered a prognostic predictor in chronic lymphocytic leukemia? Clin Lymphoma Myeloma Leuk 2013;13:441–6.
32. Myint H, Copplestone JA, Orchard J, et al. Fludarabine-related autoimmune haemolytic anaemia in patients with chronic lymphocytic leukaemia. Br J Haematol 1995;91:341–4.
33. Jeffries M, Hamadeh F, Aberle T, et al. Haemolytic anaemia in a multi-ethnic cohort of lupus patients: a clinical and serological perspective. Lupus 2008;17: 739–43.
34. Hochberg MC. Updating the American College of Rheumatology revised criteria for the classification of systemic lupus erythematosus. Arthritis Rheum 1997;40: 1725.
35. Seve P, Bourdillon L, Sarrot-Reynauld F, et al. Autoimmune hemolytic anemia and common variable immunodeficiency: a case-control study of 18 patients. Medicine (Baltimore) 2008;87:177–84.
36. Worlledge SM. Immune drug-induced haemolytic anemias. Semin Hematol 1969; 6:181–200.
37. Zantek ND, Koepsell SA, Tharp DR Jr, et al. The direct antiglobulin test: a critical step in the evaluation of hemolysis. Am J Hematol 2012;87:707–9.
38. Conley CL, Lippman SM, Ness P. Autoimmune hemolytic anemia with reticulocytopenia. A medical emergency. JAMA 1980;244:1688–90.
39. Allgood JW, Chaplin H Jr. Idiopathic acquired autoimmune hemolytic anemia. A review of forty-seven cases treated from 1955 through 1965. Am J Med 1967;43: 254–73.
40. Barcellini W, Fattizzo B, Zaninoni A, et al. Clinical heterogeneity and predictors of outcome in primary autoimmune hemolytic anemia: a GIMEMA study of 308 patients. Blood 2014;124:2930–6.
41. Chertkow G, Dacie JV. Results of splenectomy in auto-immune haemolytic anaemia. Br J Haematol 1956;2:237–49.
42. Birgens H, Frederiksen H, Hasselbalch HC, et al. A phase III randomized trial comparing glucocorticoid monotherapy versus glucocorticoid and rituximab in patients with autoimmune haemolytic anaemia. Br J Haematol 2013;163:393–9.
43. Moyo VM, Smith D, Brodsky I, et al. High-dose cyclophosphamide for refractory autoimmune hemolytic anemia. Blood 2002;100:704–6.
44. Wouters D, Stephan F, Strengers P, et al. C1-esterase inhibitor concentrate rescues erythrocytes from complement-mediated destruction in autoimmune hemolytic anemia. Blood 2013;121:1242–4.
45. Chao MP, Hong J, Kunder C, et al. Refractory warm IgM-mediated autoimmune hemolytic anemia associated with Churg-Strauss syndrome responsive to eculizumab and rituximab. Am J Hematol 2014;90:78–81.
46. Shi J, Rose EL, Singh A, et al. TNT003, an inhibitor of the serine protease C1s, prevents complement activation induced by cold agglutinins. Blood 2014;123: 4015–22.

Cold Agglutinin-Mediated Autoimmune Hemolytic Anemia

Sigbjørn Berentsen, MD, PhD[a],*, Ulla Randen, MD, PhD[b],
Geir E. Tjønnfjord, MD, PhD[c]

KEYWORDS

- Autoimmune hemolytic anemia • B lymphocytes • Cold agglutinin
- Cold agglutinin disease • Cold agglutinin syndrome • Complement
- Lymphoproliferative disorders • Therapy

KEY POINTS

- Primary chronic cold agglutinin disease (CAD) is a clonal lymphoproliferative disorder and a distinct clinicopathologic entity.
- Secondary cold agglutinin syndrome (CAS) occasionally complicates specific infections or aggressive lymphomas.
- In both CAD and CAS, hemolysis is entirely complement dependent.
- Hemolysis is predominantly extravascular, mediated by the classical complement pathway.
- Targeting the pathogenic B-lymphocyte clone has resulted in successful therapy for CAD. Complement modulation is promising in specific situations, but has to be further developed and documented before clinical use.

INTRODUCTION

Cold antibody types account for approximately 25% of autoimmune hemolytic anemias (AIHA) and are classified as shown in **Box 1**.[1–3] Most cold-reactive autoantibodies are cold agglutinins (CA). CA are antibodies that bind to erythrocyte surface antigens at low temperatures, causing agglutination and complement-mediated hemolysis. We review the etiology, pathogenesis, clinical features, and therapy of CA-mediated AIHA, highlighting the role of complement involvement. Paroxysmal cold hemoglobinuria is not addressed, because it is described elsewhere in this issue and the involved autoantibodies are not agglutinins.

The authors have nothing to disclose.
[a] Department of Medicine, Haugesund Hospital, Karmsundgata 120, Haugesund NO-5504, Norway; [b] Department of Pathology, Oslo University Hospital, Ullernchausseen 70, NO-0310 Oslo, Norway; [c] Department of Haematology, Oslo University Hospital, Institute of Clinical Medicine, University of Oslo, Sognsvannsveien 20, NO-0372 Oslo, Norway
* Corresponding author.
E-mail address: sigbjorn.berentsen@haugnett.no

Hematol Oncol Clin N Am 29 (2015) 455–471
http://dx.doi.org/10.1016/j.hoc.2015.01.002
0889-8588/15/$ – see front matter © 2015 Elsevier Inc. All rights reserved.

Box 1
Autoimmune hemolytic anemia

Warm antibody type

  Primary

  Secondary

Cold antibody type

  Primary chronic cold agglutinin disease

  Secondary cold agglutinin syndrome

    Associated with malignant disease

    Acute, infection associated

  Paroxysmal cold hemoglobinuria

Mixed cold and warm antibody type

Data from Refs.[1–3]

COLD AGGLUTININS

Cold hemagglutination was first described in 1903.[4] CA are determined semiquantitatively by their titer, based on their ability to agglutinate erythrocytes at 4°C.[5] A proportion of the adult population has demonstrable CA in serum without any evidence of hemolysis or disease; a frequency of positive screening tests at 0.3% has been reported in a cohort of patients with nonrelated disorders.[6,7] These normally occurring CA are polyclonal and are found in low titers, usually below 64 and rarely exceeding 256.[6,8] In 172 consecutive individuals with monoclonal immunoglobulin (Ig)M in serum, on the other hand, significant CA activity was found in 8.5% with titers between 512 and 65,500, and all individuals with detectable CA had hemolysis.[9] Thus, monoclonal CA are generally far more pathogenic than polyclonal CA.

The thermal amplitude is defined as the highest temperature at which the CA reacts with the antigen. In general, the pathogenicity of CA depends more on the thermal amplitude than on the titer.[10–12] The normally occurring CA have low thermal amplitudes. If the thermal amplitude exceeds 28°C or 30°C, erythrocytes agglutinate in the circulation in acral parts of the body, even at mild ambient temperatures and, often, complement fixation and complement-mediated hemolysis ensues. CA should not be confused with cryoglobulins. In rare cases, however, the cryoprotein can have both CA and cryoglobulin properties.[13,14]

Most CAs are directed against the Ii blood group system.[5,15] The I and i antigens are carbohydrate macromolecules and the density of these antigens on the erythrocyte surface are inversely proportional. Neonatal red blood cells almost exclusively express the i antigen, whereas the I antigen predominates in individuals of 18 months of age and older.[16] Therefore, CA with anti-I specificity are more pathogenic in children as well as adults than those specific for the i antigen. Occasionally, CA show specificity against the erythrocyte surface protein antigen designated Pr and such CA can be highly pathogenic.[17,18] Other specificities have been reported, but are probably very rare.[8] More than 90% of pathogenic CA are of the IgM class and these IgM macromolecules can be pentameric or hexameric.[19–21] Hexameric IgM is more pathogenic than pentameric IgM.[20]

The terms *cold agglutinin disease* (CAD) and *cold agglutinin syndrome* (CAS) have been used in the literature in a rather random way. We should distinguish, however, between these concepts. CAD is a well-defined clinicopathologic entity, as shown herein and should be called a disease, not syndrome.[3,22] The term CAS is appropriate for the secondary CA-mediated syndrome occasionally complicating specific infections or malignancies.

CHRONIC COLD AGGLUTININ DISEASE
Epidemiology

Primary CAD has been reported to account for about 15% of AIHA.[1,2] In Scandinavia, the prevalence has been estimated to 16 per million inhabitants and the incidence rate to 1 per million per year, which is probably a slight underestimation.[21] There seems to be a slight female preponderance with a male-to-female ratio of approximately 0.6:1. In the same population-based, descriptive study, the median age of the patients was 76 years (range, 51–96) and the median age at onset of clinical symptoms 67 years (30–92).[21]

Clonality and Histopathology

The first monoclonal protein ever described was a CA from a patient with CAD[23]; early studies showed that, in most patients, the CA was monoclonal IgM with kappa light chain restriction.[24,25] In a more recent study of 86 patients, the CA was found to be monoclonal IgM-kappa in more than 90% of patients.[21] Monoclonal IgG, IgA, or lambda light chain restriction were rare findings.[21] In 6% of the patients, monoclonal Ig could not be detected despite otherwise typical primary CAD. This is probably a matter of sensitivity. Furthermore, 90% of patients in whom flow cytometry of bone marrow aspirate had been performed, had a clonal expansion of kappa-positive B cells.[21] The CA in CAD are almost always specific for the I antigen and show restriction to the *IGHV4-34* gene segment.[5,22,26] These findings have led to the conclusion that patients with CAD must have a clonal B-cell lymphoproliferative disorder, which has not been elucidated fully until recent years.

Two large, retrospective studies of consecutive patients found signs of a bone marrow clonal lymphoproliferation in most patients.[21,27] Undoubtedly, this majority represents the same group of patients that has traditionally been diagnosed with "primary" or "idiopathic" CAD. Within each series, however, the individual hematologic and histologic diagnoses showed a striking heterogeneity.[21,27] In 1 series, lymphoplasmacytic lymphoma was the most frequent finding, whereas marginal zone lymphoma, unclassified clonal lymphoproliferation, and reactive lymphocytosis were also reported frequently.[21]

The explanation for this perceived heterogeneity was probably revealed by a recent study in which bone marrow biopsy samples and aspirates from 54 patients with CAD were reexamined systematically by a group of lymphoma pathologists using a standardized panel of morphologic, immunohistochemical, flow cytometric, and molecular methods.[22] The bone marrow findings in these patients were consistent with a surprisingly homogeneous disorder termed 'primary CA-associated lymphoproliferative disease' by the authors and distinct from lymphoplasmacytic lymphoma, marginal zone lymphoma, and other previously recognized lymphoma entities (**Fig. 1**). The MYD88 L265P somatic mutation, typical for lymphoplasmacytic lymphoma, could not be detected in any of 15 samples from patients with CAD tested for this mutation, even though a sensitive, polymerase chain reaction-based method was used.[22,28,29]

Complement-Mediated Hemolysis

Cooling of blood during passage through acral parts of the circulation allows CA to bind to erythrocytes and cause agglutination (**Fig. 2**). Being a strong complement

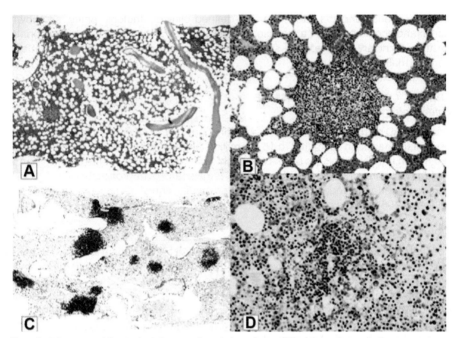

Fig. 1. Primary cold agglutinin-associated lymphoproliferative disease. Bone marrow trephine biopsy showing intraparenchymatous nodular lymphoid lesions (*A* and *B*; stain: hematoxylin and eosin; original magnification, ×40 and ×200, respectively). Immunoperoxidase staining for CD20 highlights clonal B-cell infiltration (*C*; original magnification, ×200). Mast cells are not usually discerned around the lymphoid lesions (*D*; stain: Giemsa; original magnification, ×200). (*From* Randen U, Troen G, Tierens A, et al. Primary cold agglutinin-associated lymphoproliferative disease: a B-cell lymphoma of the bone marrow distinct from lymphoplasmacytic lymphoma. Haematologica 2014;99(3):499, with permission.)

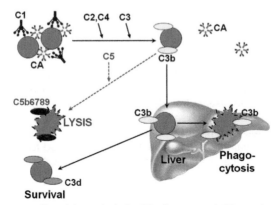

Fig. 2. Complement-mediated hemolysis in CA disease and CA syndrome. *Black arrows*, major pathway; *dotted arrows*, minor pathway; C, complement protein; CA, cold agglutinin.

activator, antigen-bound IgM CA on the cell surface binds complement protein 1 (C1) and thereby initiates the classical complement pathway.[30–32] C1 esterase activates C4 and C2, generating C3 convertase, which results in the cleavage of C3 to C3a and C3b. Upon returning to central parts of the body with a temperature of 37°C, IgM CA detaches from the cell surface, allowing agglutinated cells to separate, while C3b remains bound. A proportion of the C3b-coated erythrocytes is sequestered by macrophages of the reticuloendothelial system, mainly Kupffer cells in the liver. On the surface of the surviving red blood cells, C3b is cleaved, leaving high numbers of C3d molecules on the cell surface. These mechanisms explain why the monospecific direct antiglobulin test (DAT) is strongly positive for C3d in patients with CA-mediated hemolysis and, in the majority, negative for IgM and IgG.[21]

Complement activation may proceed beyond the C3b formation step, resulting in C5 activation, formation of the membrane attack complex (MAC), and intravascular hemolysis. Owing to surface-bound regulatory proteins such as CD55 and CD59, however, the complement activation is usually not sufficient to produce clinically significant activation of the terminal complement pathway. The major mechanism of hemolysis in stable disease, therefore, is the extravascular destruction of C3b-coated erythrocytes.[30,32,33] Obviously, however, C5-mediated intravascular hemolysis does occur in severe acute exacerbations and in some profoundly hemolytic patients, as evidenced by the observation of hemoglobinuria in 15% of the patients,[27] the rather frequent finding of hemosiderinuria (M. J. Stone 2014, personal communication) and the beneficial effect of C5 inhibition in at least occasional patients.[34]

Clinical Features

By definition, all patients with CAD have hemolysis, but occasional patients are not anemic because the hemolysis is fully compensated. Most patients, however, have manifest hemolytic anemia. The anemia can be more severe than often stated in textbooks and review articles. Of 16 patients described in an early publication, 5 had hemoglobin (Hgb) levels below 7.0 g/dL and 1 had levels below 5.0 g/dL.[25] Hgb levels ranged from 4.5 g/dL to normal in a more recent, population-based, descriptive study of 86 Norwegian patients.[21] The median Hgb level was 8.9 g/dL and the lower tertile was 8.0 g/dL. Hemoglobinuria has been reported in at least 15% of the patients.[27] About 50% of the patients are considered transfusion dependent for shorter or longer periods during the course of the disease.[21,27] In many patients, therefore, CAD is not an indolent disease in terms of clinical symptoms and quality of life.

Approximately 90% of the patients experience cold-induced acrocyanosis and/or Raynaud phenomenon.[21] The circulatory symptoms can range from slight to disabling. In cool climates, characteristic seasonal variations in the severity of hemolytic anemia have been well-documented.[35] In at least 70% of patients, exacerbation of hemolytic anemia is also triggered by febrile infections or major trauma.[21,36,37] The explanation for this paradoxical exacerbation is that, during steady-state CAD, most patients are complement depleted with low levels of C3 and, in particular, C4. During acute phase reactions, C3 and C4 are replete and complement-induced hemolysis increases.[5,37]

The median overall survival of patients with CAD has been estimated to be 12.5 years, similar to that of a general age- and sex-matched population.[21] Transformation of the lymphoproliferative bone marrow disorder to aggressive lymphoma is rare, probably with a cumulative rate of 3% to 4%. The clinical course is unpredictable; patients can experience either worsening or improvement with time, quite stable disease or, occasionally, a shift in the respective clinical manifestations.[21,36]

Diagnosis

The diagnosis of CAD should be based on history and clinical findings, assessment of hemolysis, the DAT pattern, and the CA titer. An additional electrophoretic, histopathologic, and flow cytometric workup should always be done, but demonstration of clonality may sometimes be difficult and is not absolutely required for diagnosis in the routine clinical setting. **Table 1** shows the diagnostic criteria.[3,38] Correct handling of samples as indicated in **Table 1** is essential for reliable assessment.[3,38]

Nonpharmacologic Management

Given that drug therapy has been largely ineffective until the last 10 to 15 years, counseling has been considered the mainstay of management.[25,39] Owing to the high thermal amplitude of the CA, however, the physiologic cooling of the blood in the peripheral vessels is usually sufficient to cause hemolysis and circulatory symptoms even at mild ambient temperatures.[10,21]

Most authors agree that patients should avoid cold exposure, particularly of the head, face, and extremities.[25,39–41] Those living in cool climates often, even before the diagnosis has been established, tell the physician that they use warm clothing and, in many cases, stay indoors during winter. Many patients experience improvement of Hgb levels and circulatory symptoms when temporarily relocating to a warmer climate during the cold season, but severely symptomatic CAD does exist even in the subtropics. Any liquids infused should be prewarmed, and surgery under hypothermic conditions should be avoided or specific precautions undertaken.

Erythrocyte transfusions can be given safely, provided that appropriate precautions are undertaken.[40,42] In contrast with the compatibility problems encountered in warm

Table 1
Diagnostic criteria for primary chronic CA disease

Level	Criteria	Procedures and Comments
Required for diagnosis	Chronic hemolysis	
	Polyspecific DAT positive	
	Monospecific DAT strongly positive for C3d	DAT is usually negative for IgG, but occasionally weakly positive
	CA titer ≥64 at 4°C	Blood specimen must be kept at 37°C–38°C from sampling until serum is removed from the clot
	No overt malignant disease	Clinical assessment; radiology as required
Confirmatory but not required for diagnosis	Monoclonal IgMκ in serum (or, rarely, IgG, IgA, or λ phenotype)	Serum must be obtained as for CA titer
		Immunofixation should be done even if no band is visible on electrophoresis
	Cellular κ/λ ratio >3.5 (or, rarely, <0.9) in B-lymphocyte population	Flow cytometry in bone marrow aspirate
	CA-associated lymphoproliferative bone marrow disorder by histology	Trephine biopsy

Abbreviations: CA, cold agglutinin; DAT, direct antiglobulin test; Ig, immunoglobulin.
Data from Berentsen S, Tjonnfjord GE. Diagnosis and treatment of cold agglutinin mediated autoimmune hemolytic anemia. Blood Rev 2012;26(3):107–15; and Berentsen S, Beiske K, Tjonnfjord GE. Primary chronic cold agglutinin disease: an update on pathogenesis, clinical features and therapy. Hematology 2007;12(5):361–70.

antibody AIHA, it is usually easy to find compatible donor erythrocytes, and screening tests for irregular blood group antibodies are most often negative. Antibody screening and, if required, compatibility tests should be performed at 37°C. The patient and, in particular, the extremity chosen for infusion should be kept warm, and the use of an in-line blood warmer is recommended.[39,40,42] Failure to adhere to required precautions has resulted in dismal or, very rarely, even fatal outcomes.[42,43] Because complement proteins can exacerbate hemolysis, transfusion of blood products with a high plasma content should probably be avoided.[37]

Based on theoretical considerations and clinical experience, plasmapheresis is regarded an efficient "first-aid" in acute situations or before surgery requiring hypothermia, because almost all IgM is located intravascularly.[44] Such remissions, however, are very short lived and concomitant specific therapy should usually be initiated.[39,42] Complement inhibitor-based alternative approaches to this situation are discussed elsewhere in this article. Given that the extravascular hemolysis predominantly takes place in the liver, splenectomy should not be used for the treatment of CAD. Three splenectomized patients were registered in our population-based descriptive study; none of them responded.[21] Improvement after splenectomy has been reported occasionally among the rare patients with CAD mediated by an IgG CA instead of IgM.[45]

Unspecific Immunosuppression and Supportive Drug Therapy

In textbooks and review articles, it is often postulated that typical patients with CAD are just slightly anemic and do not require pharmacologic therapy. Based on the Hgb levels and clinical features described herein, this holds true for a minority only. In Norway as well as the United States, drug therapy had been attempted in 70% to 80% of unselected patients studied in 2 relatively large, retrospective series.[21,27]

In contrast with warm antibody AIHA, corticosteroids are of little or no value in CAD.[21,27,39,40,46] Monotherapy with alkylating agents has shown some beneficial effect on laboratory parameters and clinical improvement has been observed.[47,48] The clinical response rates, however, are probably in the same low order of magnitude as for corticosteroids.[21] In 2 small series of patients treated with interferon-α or low-dose cladribine, these drugs were not shown to be useful, although some conflicting data do exist for interferon-α.[49–51] Only a few patients treated with azathioprine have been reported; none of them responded.[21]

Exacerbations precipitated by febrile illnesses should warrant immediate treatment of any bacterial infection.[37,38] Supportive therapy with erythropoietin or its analogs seems to be used widely in North America, but less often in Scandinavia and Western Europe. No studies have been published to support or discourage its use. Although poorly documented, folic acid supplements have often been recommended.[39]

Therapies Directed at the Pathogenic B-Cell Clone

The relative success in therapy for CAD during the last 10 to 12 years has been achieved by targeting the pathogenic B-cell clone.[52–54]

Rituximab monotherapy

Monotherapy with rituximab 375 mg/m² weekly for 4 weeks was studied in 2 prospective, uncontrolled trials of 37 and 20 treatment courses.[55,56] The response criteria used in the Norwegian study are shown in **Table 2**; similar strict definitions were used in the Danish study. The overall response rate was 54% and 45% in the 2 trials. With the exception of 1 complete response (CR) observed in the Norwegian trial, all remissions were partial responses (PR). Ten patients were treated for relapse after previously

Table 2
CAD: response criteria used in clinical trials

Response Level	Definition
Complete response (CR)	Absence of anemia No signs of hemolysis Disappearance of clinical symptoms of CAD No monoclonal serum protein No signs of clonal lymphoproliferation as assessed by bone marrow histology, immunohistochemistry and flow cytometry
Partial response (PR)	A stable increase in hemoglobin levels by $\geq$2.0 g/dL or to the normal range A reduction of serum IgM levels by $\geq$50% of the initial level or to the normal range Improvement of clinical symptoms Transfusion independence
No response (NR)	Any outcome not meeting the criteria for CR or PR

Abbreviations: CAD, cold agglutinin disease.
Data from Berentsen S, Ulvestad E, Gjertsen BT, et al. Rituximab for primary chronic cold agglutinin disease: a prospective study of 37 courses of therapy in 27 patients. Blood 2004;103(8):2925–8; and Berentsen S, Randen U, Vagan AM, et al. High response rate and durable remissions following fludarabine and rituximab combination therapy for chronic cold agglutinin disease. Blood 2010;116(17):3180–4.

having received rituximab therapy and 6 of them responded to a second course. In our study, the responders achieved a median increase in Hgb levels of 4.0 g/dL. We found a median time to response of 1.5 months (range, 0.5–4.0) and median response duration of 11 months (range, 2–42).[55]

In a population-based study of 86 unselected Norwegian patients with primary CAD, 40 patients were reported to have received rituximab monotherapy.[21] As far as permitted by available data, the same response criteria as previously published (see **Table 2**) were used for the retrospective analysis. Twenty-three patients (58%) were found to have responded; 2 (5%) achieving CR and 21 (53%) PR.[21] Responses had been observed after a second and even a third course of rituximab in patients who had relapsed after previous therapy. A descriptive, retrospective, single-center study from the United States noted an 83% overall response rate to single agent rituximab, although the response criteria were not specified.[27] These findings confirm the essential results of the prospective studies; rituximab monotherapy is an efficient treatment for primary CAD. CR is uncommon, however; the median response duration is relatively short and the number of nonresponders is considerable.

Adverse effects were few and tolerable in all 4 series.[21,27,55,56] Data from rituximab maintenance in patients with follicular lymphoma indicate that even prolonged or repeated administration of this monoclonal antibody is safe with regard to infections.[57] Very rare cases of progressive multifocal leukoencephalopathy and hepatitis B reactivation have been reported, however, in patients receiving rituximab for polyclonal autoimmune disorders.[58] Any causal associations are uncertain because of concomitant immunosuppressive therapies and immune dysregulation as part of the autoimmune disease itself.

Fludarabine and rituximab combination therapy

The safety and efficacy of combination therapy with fludarabine and rituximab was studied in a prospective, uncontrolled trial in 29 patients aged 39 to 87 years (median, 73) with primary CAD requiring treatment.[59] The participants received rituximab 375 mg/m^2 on days 1, 29, 57, and 85 and fludarabine orally 40 mg/m^2 on days 1 through 5, 29 through 34, 57 through 61, and 85 through 89. We used the same response criteria as published previously (see **Table 2**). Twenty-two patients (76%) responded, 6 (21%) achieving CR and 16 (55%) achieving PR. Among 10 patients nonresponsive to rituximab monotherapy, CR was observed in 1 patient and PR in 6. Median increase in Hgb level was 3.1 g/dL in the responders and 4.0 g/dL among those who achieved CR. Median time to response was 4.0 months. The lower quartile of response duration was not reached after 33 months, and estimated median response duration was more than 66 months (**Fig. 3**).

Grade 3 and 4 hematologic toxicity occurred in 12 patients (41%); neutropenia accounted for all cases of grade 4 toxicity. Seventeen patients (59%) had infection grade 1 through 3, which was successfully treated in all except for 1 elderly, frail nonresponder who died of pneumonia 9 months after treatment. Cotrimoxazol or anti-viral prophylaxis was not given routinely. Infection grade 4 or *Pneumocystis jirovecii* pneumonia did not occur, but 3 patients (10%) experienced herpes zoster reactivation. Transient exacerbation of hemolytic anemia was seen in 3 patients (10%). All 3 were found to have exacerbation of CAD precipitated by infection,[37] whereas fludarabine-induced warm antibody AIHA was not observed. Nearly one-half of patients had their doses of fludarabine reduced because of hematologic toxicity.[59]

Comparison of nonrandomized trials should be undertaken with care. Nonetheless, the baseline data reported in the fludarabine–rituximab trial matched well with those described in the trials of rituximab monotherapy.[55,56,59] The response criteria (see **Table 2**) were identical in the 2 Norwegian studies and very similar to those used in the Danish monotherapy trial. The 76% response rate and more than 66 months estimated response duration achieved by using fludarabine and rituximab in combination,

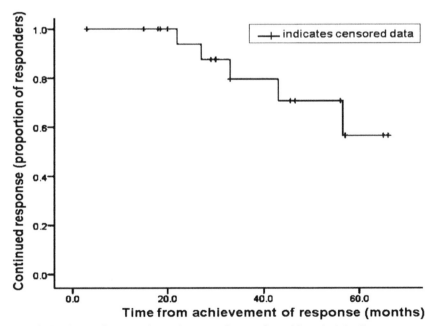

Fig. 3. Fludarabin and rituximab combination therapy for cold agglutinin disease: response duration. (*From* Berentsen S, Randen U, Vagan AM, et al. High response rate and durable remissions following fludarabine and rituximab combination therapy for chronic cold agglutinin disease. Blood 2010;116(17):3182, with permission.)

therefore, compare favorably with the 45% to 54% response rate and 11 months response duration observed after monotherapy with rituximab. Furthermore, CR was achieved in 21% of the patients after the combination therapy, whereas remissions are rarely complete after rituximab monotherapy. Ten patients acted as their own controls by receiving the combination after rituximab single agent therapy had failed.[59] With the achievement of 1 CR and 6 PR in this subgroup, the combination has been shown to be effective even in patients nonresponsive to monotherapy with rituximab.

Given the relative toxicity of the fludarabin–rituximab combination, the therapeutic potential should be weighed carefully against the short-term risks, particularly in very old and comorbid patients. We found, however, no association between adverse events and age itself.[59] The study was not designed to assess the risk of secondary hematologic malignancies. Although not specific to purine nucleoside analogs, late-occurring acute myelogenous leukemia and myelodysplastic syndromes have been observed after fludarabine-based therapy for Waldenström's macroglobulinemia.[60] This concern should not be prohibitive to the use of rituximab and fludarabine in combination, but rather lead to a balanced, individualized consideration of benefit versus long-term risk, particularly in the younger patients.

Other therapy targeting the clonal B cells
Favorable results of combination therapy with bendamustine and rituximab have been reported in 1 single patient, but no systematic study has been published to date.[61] Improvement after bortezomib-based therapy or a cyclophosphamide-containing combination has been described in single case reports.[14,62]

Future Perspectives: Complement-Directed Therapy?
Eculizumab, a monoclonal anti-C5 antibody, is a powerful therapeutic agent in paroxysmal nocturnal hemoglobinuria (PNH). In PNH, however, the predominant route of complement-mediated hemolysis is the intravascular cell destruction caused by activation of the terminal complement pathway, starting with C5 cleavage. Nevertheless, eculizumab therapy did produce major improvement of CAD according to 1 single case report.[9] Further studies may elucidate the representativeness of this observation.

The only classical pathway inhibitor currently available for clinical use is plasma-derived or recombinant C1-esterase inhibitor (C1-INH), which is approved for the treatment of hereditary angioedema (HAE). Although not a complement-mediated disorder, HAE is caused by lack or deficiency of endogenous C1-INH and replacement therapy is well-established.[63] In AIHA, on the other hand, endogenous C1-INH production is normal, indicating that physiologic concentrations of the inhibitor will not block complement-mediated hemolysis. Pharmacologic doses of C1-INH did, however, result in improvement in a well-described case of severe warm antibody AIHA.[64]

A recent in vitro study tested the effects of TNT003, a mouse monoclonal antibody targeting C1, on CA-induced complement activity against human erythrocytes.[30] This antibody has specificity for the complement serine protease C1s. Using CA samples from 40 patients with CAD, the authors found that TNT003 prevented CA-induced hemolysis. TNT003 also blocked deposition of C3 fragments on the erythrocytes at the same concentration of antibody that stopped hemolysis. Furthermore, the inhibition of C1s resulted in prevention of in vitro erythrophagocytosis by a phagocytic cell line. The monoclonal antibody also inhibited the CA-induced, classical pathway-driven generation of anaphylotoxins C4a, C3a, and C5a. Interestingly, CA from only 1 patient sample out of 40 was able to directly induce MAC-mediated hemolysis. These findings reveal an interesting potential for using a corresponding humanized antibody for the treatment of CAD and, in addition, support the existing view that complement activity in CAD terminates before activation of the terminal pathway in most patients.[30,65,66]

Small molecule peptide inhibitors of the classical complement pathway are also of potential interest.[67] Peptide inhibitor of C1 (PIC1) is a recently described class of such molecules that targets C1q, blocking the activation of associated serine proteases (C1s–C1r–C1r–C1s) and subsequent downstream complement activation.[68] These molecules have also been shown to inhibit the lectin pathway.[68] PIC1 has been studied in acute hemolytic transfusion reaction in animal models but, so far, not in CA-related experiments. Another interesting low-molecular-weight inhibitor is compstatin Cp40, a peptide that blocks cleavage of C3. Although no specific data have been published for CA-induced hemolysis, compstatin has been found to efficiently prevent in vitro lysis of red blood cells from PNH patients.[69]

Given that the complement system is an essential part of the innate immune system, it is important to ask whether complement modulation will be too dangerous. Regarding eculizumab therapy in PNH, we know that the risk of severe infection after C5 inhibition is negligible, provided that the patients can be efficiently protected against meningococci.[70] Modulation at the C3 level may carry a much greater risk because efficient inhibition of C3 completely blocks complement activation beyond this level, whether initiated by the classical, alternative, or lectin pathway.[66,69]

Interestingly, the still more proximal blockade at the C1 level achieved by TNT003 selectively affects the classical pathway as required for control of hemolysis in CAD, whereas the lectin and alternative pathways remain intact. Probably, therefore, these pathways will still enable the system to generate anaphylotoxins C3a and C5a in response to microbial stimuli, even though the production of these anaphylotoxins induced by the classical pathway will be blocked.[30] Although this selectivity may, theoretically, reduce the risk of infection, careful studies are required to address this issue. Finally, temporary complement inhibition in acute situations (eg, acute phase reaction–induced exacerbation or preoperative management) may be expected to be less dangerous than long-term therapy.

SECONDARY COLD AGGLUTININ SYNDROME
Mycoplasma Infection

Mycoplasma pneumoniae pneumonia is the most frequent cause of secondary CAS and has been reported to account for 8% of the cases of AIHA.[2] Patients with *M pneumoniae* infections produce CA as part of the physiologic immune response, but most of them do not develop hemolytic anemia. Occasionally, however, production of high-titer, high-thermal amplitude CA can result in hemolysis.[71–73] Among 25 patients with *Mycoplasma* infection admitted to a referral center, 6 (25%) had hemolysis, which was severe in 2 patients and mild to moderate in 4.[73] In general hospitals and the community, the frequency of hemolytic complications is obviously much lower.

In CAS caused by *Mycoplasma*, the CA are polyclonal, anti-I–specific and almost invariably of the IgM class; and titers usually range between 512 and 32,000.[72] DAT is always positive for C3d. The onset of anemia typically occurs during the second or third week after the febrile infection has started. Although the hemolytic anemia can be severe, the prognosis is generally good and the complication is self-remitting within 4 to 6 weeks.[3,72] A lethal course has been described in 1 patient.[74]

Epstein–Barr Virus Infection

CA-mediated AIHA, usually but not invariably mild, occasionally complicates infectious mononucleosis with confirmed Epstein–Barr virus (EBV) etiology.[3,75–77]

Compared with *M pneumoniae* pneumonia, EBV is an infrequent cause of AIHA, accounting for approximately 1% of cases.[1,2] Conversely, the frequency of clinically significant hemolysis in EBV infections is unknown, but probably low.[3,76] The CA are polyclonal and almost invariably specific for the i antigen.[75,77]

Other Infections

Several series and case reports have described transient CAS mediated by anti-i autoantibodies after cytomegalovirus infection.[77,78] Rarely, CA-mediated hemolysis has been reported in adenovirus infections, influenza A, varicella, rubella, *Legionella pneumophilica* pneumonia, listeriosis, and pneumonia caused by *Chlamydia* species. Severe CAS with a prolonged course and cryoglobulin activity of the CA has been observed following *Escherichia coli* lung infection. Autoantibody specificities in these rare cases have included anti-I, anti-i, and anti-Pr.[3]

Aggressive Lymphoma

Among 295 consecutive individuals with AIHA described by Dacie,[2] 7 patients (2.4%) were classified as having CAS secondary to malignancies. Thus, CAS secondary to overt malignant disease is far more uncommon than primary CAD. The best documentation for a clinically malignant disease resulting in CAS has been provided in aggressive non-Hodgkin lymphoma.[79–81] CA found in such patients are usually monoclonal and anti-I–specific but, unlike CA in CAD, the light chain restriction can be lambda as well as kappa.[79]

Nonlymphatic Malignancies

Systematic series as well as case reports have described secondary CAS in a variety of other malignancies, including carcinomas, sarcomas, metastatic melanoma, and myeloproliferative disorders.[1–3] Some of these associations are probably real, whereas in other examples the documentation and association may be questioned, as extensively discussed elsewhere.[3]

Therapy for Secondary Cold Agglutinin Syndrome

For obvious reasons, treatment of the underlying disease is important when possible. In curable malignancies such as aggressive lymphoma, achieving complete remission is usually accompanied by resolution of the hemolytic anemia.[3,81] *M pneumoniae* pneumonia should be treated according to existing guidelines, although, owing to the time of onset of hemolysis, antibiotic therapy will often have been initiated before the hemolytic anemia manifests itself.[72] In some viral infections, causal therapy is not possible; in others, antiviral therapy is not necessary because the CAS is slight and self-remitting.

No evidence-based therapy exists for secondary CAS per se.[3] Prospective studies or well-designed retrospective series have not been published, and recommendations have been based on clinical experience, case reports, and theoretic considerations. Improvement after the administration of corticosteroids has been described in several cases.[82,83] Because spontaneous remission occurs eventually in nearly all patients; however, guidelines cannot be built on case reports. Erythrocyte transfusions can safely be given provided the same precautions are observed as in primary CAD.[3,38,42] Plasmapheresis should be considered in selected, extreme cases.[42,84]

The possibility of intervention by complement modulation is very interesting in secondary CAS, but clinical documentation is currently nonexistent. The same options as discussed for CAD may be considered for investigation.[30,34,64,65,68,69] Unlike CAD, infection-associated acute CAS only requires temporary complement inhibition during the most severe hemolysis or until spontaneous resolution occurs. In theory, therefore, the safety issues discussed for CAD may turn out to be less problematic in CAS. Ideally, the efficacy and safety of complement modulation in severe CAS should be explored in systematic series or prospective uncontrolled trials, which will have to be done at a very large, international scale to collect statistically solid data.

REFERENCES

1. Sokol RJ, Hewitt S, Stamps BK. Autoimmune haemolysis: an 18-year study of 865 cases referred to a regional transfusion centre. Br Med J (Clin Res Ed) 1981; 282(6281):2023–7.
2. Dacie J. The auto-immune haemolytic anaemias: introduction. In: Dacie J, editor. The haemolytic anaemias, vol. 3. London: Churchill Livingstone; 1992. p. 1–5.
3. Berentsen S, Tjonnfjord GE. Diagnosis and treatment of cold agglutinin mediated autoimmune hemolytic anemia. Blood Rev 2012;26(3):107–15.
4. Landsteiner K. Über Beziehungen zwischen dem Blutserum und den Körperzellen. Münch Med Wschr 1903;50:1812–4.
5. Ulvestad E, Berentsen S, Bo K, et al. Clinical immunology of chronic cold agglutinin disease. Eur J Haematol 1999;63(4):259–66.
6. Jain MD, Cabrerzio-Sanchez R, Karkouti K, et al. Seek and you shall find–but then what do you do? Cold agglutinins in cardiopulmonary bypass and a single-center experience with cold agglutinin screening before cardiac surgery. Transfus Med Rev 2013;27(2):65–73.
7. Bendix BJ, Tauscher CD, Bryant SJ, et al. Defining a reference range for cold agglutinin titers. Transfusion 2014;54(5):1294–7.
8. Dacie J. Auto-immune haemolytic anaemia (AIHA): cold-antibody syndromes II: immunochemistry and specificity of the antibodies; serum complement in autoimmune haemolytic anaemia. In: Dacie J, editor. The haemolytic anaemias, vol. 3. London: Churchill Livingstone; 1992. p. 240–95.
9. Stone MJ, McElroy YG, Pestronk A, et al. Human monoclonal macroglobulins with antibody activity. Semin Oncol 2003;30(2):318–24.
10. Hopkins C, Walters TK. Thermal amplitude test. Immunohematology 2013;29(2): 49–50.
11. Garratty G, Petz LD, Hoops JK. The correlation of cold agglutinin titrations in saline and albumin with haemolytic anaemia. Br J Haematol 1977;35(4):587–95.
12. Rosse WF, Adams JP. The variability of hemolysis in the cold agglutinin syndrome. Blood 1980;56(3):409–16.
13. Berentsen S, Bo K, Shammas FV, et al. Chronic cold agglutinin disease of the "idiopathic" type is a premalignant or low-grade malignant lymphoproliferative disease. APMIS 1997;105(5):354–62.
14. Bhattacharyya J, Mihara K, Takihara Y, et al. Successful treatment of IgM-monoclonal gammopathy of undetermined significance associated with cryoglobulinemia and cold agglutinin disease with immunochemotherapy with rituximab, fludarabine, and cyclophosphamide. Ann Hematol 2012;91(5):797–9.
15. Issitt PD. I blood group system and its relationship to disease. J Med Lab Technol 1968;25(1):1–6.
16. Marsh WL. Anti-i: a cold antibody defining the Ii relationship in human red cells. Br J Haematol 1961;7:200–9.
17. Silberstein LE, Robertson GA, Harris AC, et al. Etiologic aspects of cold agglutinin disease: evidence for cytogenetically defined clones of lymphoid cells and the demonstration that an anti-Pr cold autoantibody is derived from a chromosomally aberrant B cell clone. Blood 1986;67(6):1705–9.

18. Brain MC, Ruether B, Valentine K, et al. Life-threatening hemolytic anemia due to an autoanti-Pr cold agglutinin: evidence that glycophorin A antibodies may induce lipid bilayer exposure and cation permeability independent of agglutination. Transfusion 2010;50(2):292–301.

19. Harboe M, Deverill J. Immunochemical properties of cold haemagglutinins. Scand J Haematol 1964;61:223–37.

20. Hughey CT, Brewer JW, Colosia AD, et al. Production of IgM hexamers by normal and autoimmune B cells: implications for the physiologic role of hexameric IgM. J Immunol 1998;161(8):4091–7.

21. Berentsen S, Ulvestad E, Langholm R, et al. Primary chronic cold agglutinin disease: a population based clinical study of 86 patients. Haematologica 2006; 91(4):460–6.

22. Randen U, Troen G, Tierens A, et al. Primary cold agglutinin-associated lymphoproliferative disease: a B-cell lymphoma of the bone marrow distinct from lymphoplasmacytic lymphoma. Haematologica 2014;99(3):497–504.

23. Christenson WN, Dacie JV, Croucher BE, et al. Electrophoretic studies on sera containing high-titre cold haemagglutinins: identification of the antibody as the cause of an abnormal gamma 1 peak. Br J Haematol 1957;3(3):262–75.

24. Harboe M, van Furth R, Schubothe H, et al. Exclusive occurrence of K chains in isolated cold haemagglutinins. Scand J Haematol 1965;2(3):259–66.

25. Schubothe H. The cold hemagglutinin disease. Semin Hematol 1966;3(1):27–47.

26. Pascual V, Victor K, Spellerberg M, et al. VH restriction among human cold agglutinins. The VH4-21 gene segment is required to encode anti-I and anti-i specificities. J Immunol 1992;149(7):2337–44.

27. Swiecicki PL, Hegerova LT, Gertz MA. Cold agglutinin disease. Blood 2013; 122(7):1114–21.

28. Treon SP, Xu L, Yang G, et al. MYD88 L265P somatic mutation in Waldenström's macroglobulinemia. N Engl J Med 2012;367(9):826–33.

29. Xu L, Hunter ZR, Yang G, et al. MYD88 L265P in Waldenström macroglobulinemia, immunoglobulin M monoclonal gammopathy, and other B-cell lymphoproliferative disorders using conventional and quantitative allele-specific polymerase chain reaction. Blood 2013;121(11):2051–8.

30. Shi J, Rose EL, Singh A, et al. TNT003, an inhibitor of the serine protease C1s, prevents complement activation induced by cold agglutinin disease patient autoantibodies. Blood 2014;123(26):4015–22.

31. Jonsen J, Kass E, Harboe M. Complement and complement components in acquired hemolytic anemia with high titer cold antibodies. Acta Med Scand 1961; 170:725–9.

32. Jaffe CJ, Atkinson JP, Frank MM. The role of complement in the clearance of cold agglutinin-sensitized erythrocytes in man. J Clin Invest 1976;58(4):942–9.

33. Kurlander RJ, Rosse WF, Logue GL. Quantitative influence of antibody and complement coating of red cells on monocyte-mediated cell lysis. J Clin Invest 1978; 61(5):1309–19.

34. Roth A, Huttmann A, Rother RP, et al. Long-term efficacy of the complement inhibitor eculizumab in cold agglutinin disease. Blood 2009;113(16):3885–6.

35. Lyckholm LJ, Edmond MB. Images in clinical medicine. Seasonal hemolysis due to cold-agglutinin syndrome. N Engl J Med 1996;334(7):437.

36. Ulvestad E. Paradoxical haemolysis in a patient with cold agglutinin disease. Eur J Haematol 1998;60(2):93–100.

37. Ulvestad E, Berentsen S, Mollnes TE. Acute phase haemolysis in chronic cold agglutinin disease. Scand J Immunol 2001;54(1–2):239–42.

38. Berentsen S, Beiske K, Tjonnfjord GE. Primary chronic cold agglutinin disease: an update on pathogenesis, clinical features and therapy. Hematology 2007; 12(5):361–70.
39. Dacie J. Treatment and prognosis of cold-antibody AIHA. In: Dacie J, editor. The haemolytic anaemias, vol. 3. London: Churchill Livingstone; 1992. p. 502–8.
40. Berentsen S. How I manage cold agglutinin disease. Br J Haematol 2011;153(3): 309–17.
41. Nydegger UE, Kazatchkine MD, Miescher PA. Immunopathologic and clinical features of hemolytic anemia due to cold agglutinins. Semin Hematol 1991; 28(1):66–77.
42. Rosenfield RE, Jagathambal. Transfusion therapy for autoimmune hemolytic anemia. Semin Hematol 1976;13(4):311–21.
43. Lodi G, Resca D, Reverberi R. Fatal cold agglutinin-induced haemolytic anaemia: a case report. J Med Case Rep 2010;4:252.
44. Zoppi M, Oppliger R, Althaus U, et al. Reduction of plasma cold agglutinin titers by means of plasmapheresis to prepare a patient for coronary bypass surgery. Infusionsther Transfusionsmed 1993;20(1–2):19–22.
45. Silberstein LE, Berkman EM, Schreiber AD. Cold hemagglutinin disease associated with IgG cold-reactive antibody. Ann Intern Med 1987;106(2):238–42.
46. Gertz MA. Management of cold haemolytic syndrome. Br J Haematol 2007; 138(4):422–9.
47. Worlledge SM, Brain MC, Cooper AC, et al. Immunosuppressive drugs in the treatment of autoimmune haemolytic anaemia. Proc R Soc Med 1968;61(12): 1312–5.
48. Hippe E, Jensen KB, Olesen H, et al. Chlorambucil treatment of patients with cold agglutinin syndrome. Blood 1970;35(1):68–72.
49. Berentsen S, Tjonnfjord GE, Shammas FV, et al. No response to cladribine in five patients with chronic cold agglutinin disease. Eur J Haematol 2000;65(1): 88–90.
50. Hillen HF, Bakker SJ. Failure of interferon-alpha-2b therapy in chronic cold agglutinin disease. Eur J Haematol 1994;53(4):242–3.
51. O'Connor BM, Clifford JS, Lawrence WD, et al. Alpha-interferon for severe cold agglutinin disease. Ann Intern Med 1989;111(3):255–6.
52. Berentsen S, Ulvestad E, Tjonnfjord GE. B-lymphocytes as targets for therapy in chronic cold agglutinin disease. Cardiovasc Hematol Disord Drug Targets 2007; 7(3):219–27.
53. Stone MJ. Heating up cold agglutinins. Blood 2010;116(17):3119–20.
54. Zanella A, Barcellini W. Treatment of autoimmune hemolytic anemias. Haematologica 2014;99(10):1547–54.
55. Berentsen S, Ulvestad E, Gjertsen BT, et al. Rituximab for primary chronic cold agglutinin disease: a prospective study of 37 courses of therapy in 27 patients. Blood 2004;103(8):2925–8.
56. Schollkopf C, Kjeldsen L, Bjerrum OW, et al. Rituximab in chronic cold agglutinin disease: a prospective study of 20 patients. Leuk Lymphoma 2006;47(2):253–60.
57. Ghielmini M, Schmitz SF, Cogliatti SB, et al. Prolonged treatment with rituximab in patients with follicular lymphoma significantly increases event-free survival and response duration compared with the standard weekly x 4 schedule. Blood 2004;103(12):4416–23.
58. Cooper N, Arnold DM. The effect of rituximab on humoral and cell mediated immunity and infection in the treatment of autoimmune diseases. Br J Haematol 2010;149(1):3–13.

59. Berentsen S, Randen U, Vagan AM, et al. High response rate and durable remissions following fludarabine and rituximab combination therapy for chronic cold agglutinin disease. Blood 2010;116(17):3180–4.
60. Leleu X, Tamburini J, Roccaro A, et al. Balancing risk versus benefit in the treatment of Waldenstrom's Macroglobulinemia patients with nucleoside analogue-based therapy. Clin Lymphoma Myeloma 2009;9(1):71–3.
61. Gueli A, Gottardi D, Hu H, et al. Efficacy of rituximab-bendamustine in cold agglutinin haemolytic anaemia refractory to previous chemo-immunotherapy: a case report. Blood Transfus 2013;11(2):311–4.
62. Carson KR, Beckwith LG, Mehta J. Successful treatment of IgM-mediated autoimmune hemolytic anemia with bortezomib. Blood 2010;115(4):915.
63. Bork K, Steffensen I, Machnig T. Treatment with C1-esterase inhibitor concentrate in type I or II hereditary angioedema: a systematic literature review. Allergy Asthma Proc 2013;34(4):312–27.
64. Wouters D, Stephan F, Strengers P, et al. C1-esterase inhibitor concentrate rescues erythrocytes from complement-mediated destruction in autoimmune hemolytic anemia. Blood 2013;121(7):1242–4.
65. Panicker S, Shi J, Rose E, et al. TNT009, a classical complement pathway specific inhibitor, prevents complement dependent hemolysis induced by cold agglutinin disease patient autoantibodies. 55th Meeting of the American Society of Hematology. New Orleans (LA), December 08, 2013 (Paper 64043). Available at: https://ash.confex.com/ash/2013/webprogram/Paper64043.html.
66. Berentsen S. Complement, cold agglutinins, and therapy. Blood 2014;123(26): 4010–2.
67. Larghi EL, Kaufman TS. Modulators of complement activation: a patent review (2008–2013). Expert Opin Ther Pat 2014;24(6):665–86.
68. Sharp JA, Whitley PH, Cunnion KM, et al. Peptide inhibitor of complement c1, a novel suppressor of classical pathway activation: mechanistic studies and clinical potential. Front Immunol 2014;5:406.
69. Risitano AM, Ricklin D, Huang Y, et al. Peptide inhibitors of C3 activation as a novel strategy of complement inhibition for the treatment of paroxysmal nocturnal hemoglobinuria. Blood 2014;123(13):2094–101.
70. Hillmen P, Young NS, Schubert J, et al. The complement inhibitor eculizumab in paroxysmal nocturnal hemoglobinuria. N Engl J Med 2006;355(12):1233–43.
71. Ginsberg HS. Acute hemolytic anemia in primary atypical pneumonia associated with high titer of cold agglutinins; report of a case. N Engl J Med 1946;234:826–9.
72. Dacie J. Auto-immune haemolytic anaemia (AIHA): cold-antibody syndromes III: haemolytic anaemia following mycoplasma pneumonia. In: Dacie J, editor. The haemolytic anaemias, vol. 3. London: Churchill Livingstone; 1992. p. 296–312.
73. Linz DH, Tolle SW, Elliot DL. Mycoplasma pneumoniae pneumonia. Experience at a referral center. West J Med 1984;140(6):895–900.
74. Schubothe H, Merz KP, Weber S, et al. Akute autoimmunhämolytische Anemie vom Kältenantikörpertype mit tödlichem Ausgang. Acta Haematol 1970;44(1):111–23.
75. Jenkins WJ, Koster HG, Marsh WL, et al. Infectious mononucleosis: an unsuspected source of anti-i. Br J Haematol 1965;11:480–3.
76. Luzuriaga K, Sullivan JL. Infectious mononucleosis. N Engl J Med 2010;362(21): 1993–2000.
77. Dacie J. Auto-immune haemolytic anaemia (AIHA): cold-antibody syndromes IV: haemolytic anaemia following infectious mononucleosis and other viral infections. In: Dacie J, editor. The haemolytic anaemias, vol. 3. London: Churchill Livingstone; 1992. p. 313–28.

78. Berlin BS, Chandler R, Green D. Anti-"I" antibody and hemolytic anemia associated with spontaneous cytomegalovirus mononucleosis. Am J Clin Pathol 1977; 67(5):459–61.
79. Crisp D, Pruzanski W. B-cell neoplasms with homogeneous cold-reacting antibodies (cold agglutinins). Am J Med 1982;72(6):915–22.
80. Niainle F, Hamnvik OP, Gulmann C, et al. Diffuse large B-cell lymphoma with isolated bone marrow involvement presenting with secondary cold agglutinin disease. Int J Lab Hematol 2008;30(5):444–5.
81. Dacie J. Haemolytic anaemias associated with malignant lymphomas other than Hodgkin's disease and chronic lymphocytic leukaemia (CLL). In: Dacie J, editor. The haemolytic anaemias, vol. 4. London: Churchill Livingstone; 1995. p. 27–40.
82. Chu CS, Braun SR, Yarbro JW, et al. Corticosteroid treatment of hemolytic anemia associated with Mycoplasma pneumoniae pneumonia. South Med J 1990;83(9): 1106–8.
83. Tsuruta R, Kawamura Y, Inoue T, et al. Corticosteroid therapy for hemolytic anemia and respiratory failure due to Mycoplasma pneumoniae pneumonia. Intern Med 2002;41(3):229–32.
84. Geurs F, Ritter K, Mast A, et al. Successful plasmapheresis in corticosteroid-resistant hemolysis in infectious mononucleosis: role of autoantibodies against triosephosphate isomerase. Acta Haematol 1992;88(2–3):142–6.

Paroxysmal Cold Hemoglobinuria

Satish Shanbhag, MBBS, MPH*, Jerry Spivak, MD

KEYWORDS

- Donath-Landsteiner • PCH • Autoimmune hemolytic anemia
- Coombs negative hemolysis • Syphilis

KEY POINTS

- Paroxysmal cold hemoglobinuria is a rare cause of autoimmune hemolytic anemia predominantly seen as an acute form in young children after viral illnesses and in a chronic form in some hematological malignancies and tertiary syphilis.
- Paroxysmal cold hemoglobinuria is a complement medicated intravascular hemolytic anemia associated with a biphasic antibody against the P antigen on red cells. The antibody attaches to red cells at colder temperatures and causes red cell lysis when blood recirculates to warmer parts of the body.
- Treatment for paroxysmal cold hemoglobinuria is mainly supportive and with red cell transfusion, but immunosuppressive therapy shows promise in severe cases.

INTRODUCTION

Of the types of autoimmune hemolytic anemias an adult hematologist will encounter, paroxysmal cold hemoglobinuria (PCH) is one of the rarest. PCH is a phenomenon seen not uncommonly in association with tertiary syphilis, and the advent of antibiotics has dramatically reduced the prevalence of this fascinating phenomenon in the developed world. A large majority of patients with PCH in the early twentith century had a chronic relapsing form of the disease in association with tertiary or congenital syphilis. Recurrent/relapsing episodes of intravascular hemolysis were precipitated by exposure of the body to cold temperatures, which improved on warming. In the modern era, when it is rare to find cases of advanced syphilis, PCH is seen mostly in young children, where it presents as acute hemolysis after a viral illness. It is usually nonrecurrent, with a male preponderance, and presents with a rapid onset syndrome with prompt recovery with rest, warmth, and blood transfusion support as needed.[1]

The authors have nothing to disclose.
Division of Hematology, Department of Medicine, The Johns Hopkins University School of Medicine, Suite 4500, 301 building 4940 Eastern Ave, Baltimore, MD 21224, USA
* Corresponding author.
E-mail address: sshanbh2@jhmi.edu

The mechanism of hemolysis in PCH was elucidated by Julius Donath and Karl Landsteiner in 1904. They described a 2-phase process: the antibodies responsible for the red cell breakdown were initially adsorbed on the red cells below normal body temperatures. The affected red cells were then lysed when circulating blood was warmed to normal body temperature.[2] This 2-step process, or the Donath-Landsteiner (DL) reaction, was one of the first laboratory tests invented in the investigation of autoimmune hemolytic anemias (AIHAs). The role of complement, and its essential part in the hemolytic reaction, was elucidated further in the early 1950s.[3]

MECHANISM OF HEMOLYSIS

PCH is a complement-mediated intravascular hemolytic process in which a polyclonal immunoglobulin G (IgG) autoantibody binds to the P antigen, a polysaccharide on the red cell surface of most humans.[4] This polyclonal IgG is unusual in that it reacts at cold temperatures (unlike most IgG-mediated hemolytic anemias that react at warm temperatures). The antibody attaches to the red blood cell (RBC) membrane along with the first 2 components of complement at colder temperatures (such as the extremities in cold weather). When the red cells circulate to warmer parts of the body, intravascular hemolysis occurs by activation of the complement cascade.

PCH is differentiated from cold agglutinin disease because it does not involve IgM antibodies and lacks the classic blood smear findings of red cell agglutination.

PREVALENCE AND CLINICAL PRESENTATION

There are limited population-level data on the prevalence of PCH, but most cases in the current day are children who present with a postinfectious acute hemolytic episode, which will likely never recur. Most cases are seen in children before their fifth birthday, with a male predominance.[5] In this age group, PCH was as common as warm autoimmune hemolytic anemia (AIHA) as the cause of hemolysis in the British study by Sokol and colleagues. This finding did not hold true in a more recent Italian study, which found PCH accounting for only 6% of total childhood cases of AIHA and with a male:female ratio of 5:1.[6] Another study found the prevalence of PCH to be about 32% of childhood cases of AIHA, also noting the higher prevalence in boys.[7] The prevalence of PCH is likely reflective of the sensitivity of the DL test, which can be increased by using papain enzyme-treated (as opposed to untreated) red cells to detect hemolysis.

Episodes of PCH in children are usually concurrent or appear after a viral or bacterial infection, including measles, mumps, cytomegalovirus, Epstein-Barr virus, varicella, influenza, mycoplasma, and Hemophilus influenzae.[8-11] Hemolysis is usually transient and self-limiting, but severe cases can result in acute renal failure.[12-14] The symptoms may include hemoglobinuria, rigors, chills, myalgias, nausea, fatigue, and jaundice. Other common symptoms are cough (likely from the viral infection), anorexia, headache, and loin and back pain.[15] The physical examination findings of PCH are those of anemia and icterus; because it is predominantly an intravascular hemolytic process, patients do not usually present with significant splenomegaly or adenopathy (unless there is an underlying process such as lymphoma).

Congenital or tertiary syphilis was responsible for more than 90% of cases of PCH in the early 1900s, with a chronic relapsing form of the disease especially worse during the winter. After the advent of effective antibiotic therapy and epidemiologic measures like contact tracing and screening of pregnant women, congenital and tertiary syphilis became rare entities.[16] Rarely, adults present with PCH after viral infections such as varicella.[10] Other cases of PCH in adults have been reported in association with non-Hodgkin lymphoma and myeloproliferative disorders, although the etiologic connection is unknown.[17,18]

LABORATORY TESTING

Laboratory abnormalities in PCH reflect intravascular hemolysis, presenting as a normocytic or macrocytic anemia. Reticulocytosis may be suppressed early on in the episode because the marrow has not yet had time to respond to the anemia or because of viral suppression of hematopoiesis. Unless the reticulocytes are more selectively targeted by the autoimmune antibody, most patients have a brisk reticulocytosis a few days after the hemolysis starts.[19] An elevated lactate dehydrogenase level, reduced haptoglobin, elevated free plasma hemoglobin, indirect hyperbilirubinemia, and urine hemoglobinuria and hemosiderinuria are also seen. All complement levels are usually low after hemolysis due to consumption.

Classic blood smear findings in PCH can be subtle—polychromasia is dependent on reticulocytosis after the marrow has had time to respond. Microspherocytes are usually seen but are nowhere as abundant as in warm AIHA.[20] Red cell agglutination is also limited in contrast to what is seen in cold agglutinin disease. A classic smear finding, although not seen very frequently—neutrophil erythrophagocytosis has a strong association with PCH when it is present (**Fig. 1**).[3,21–24]

Direct antiglobulin testing (DAT or direct Coomb) of the patient's serum usually does not react with the screening antisera or anti-IgG. C3 antisera can be frequently positive on DAT, although some cases are Coomb negative.

The DL test is specific for PCH; the patient's serum is cooled to 4°C to allow for fixing of complement to the P antigen on the RBC membrane. The sample is then warmed to 37°C with papain (to open up more P-antigen sites on red cells), which causes complement-mediated hemolysis. The control sample that did not get cooled and remained at 37°C should not have any hemolysis.

The indirect DL test, a variant of the indirect Coomb test, can be used when sample volume is limited or when the direct DL test is negative but the clinical suspicion for PCH is high. The patient's serum is separated, collected at 37°C, and mixed with ABO-compatible P-positive red cells. The sample is then cooled to 4°C for 1 hour followed by warming to 37°C for 30 minutes. Hemolysis in the centrifuged supernatant serum indicates a positive result, while the control serum (which is maintained at 37°C without cooling) should appear clear. The sensitivity of the test can be increased by using ABO-compatible serum as an additional source of complement to increase the rate of red cell lysis.[15]

Thermal range is the highest "cold" temperature of the primary phase at which in vitro hemolysis can still be observed in the DL test. Maximum hemolysis is usually observed when the sample is cooled to 0°C. The antibody causing acute PCH can show thermal activity up to 24°C, while in chronic PCH (eg, after syphilis), the antibody usually does not cause red cell lysis at primary incubation temperatures higher than 15°C. This in vitro test is a measure of the potency of the DL antibody; however, the antibody must bind at much higher temperatures in vivo, ranging from 30°C to 37°C within the human body.[15,25]

TREATMENT

Hemolysis in acute PCH is usually transient and self-limiting. The severity of presentation depends on the rate of hemolysis and development of anemia—supportive measures, including keeping the patient warm and avoiding any cold exposure, are essential. The red cell transfusion requirement depends on the severity of anemia

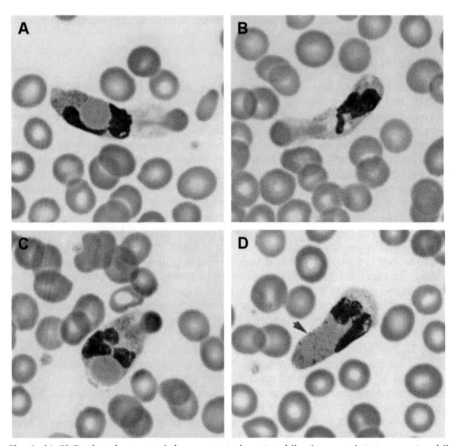

Fig. 1. (*A–D*) Erythrophagocytosis by segmented neutrophils. *Arrow* points to a neutrophil with a phagocytosed red cell in it's cytoplasm. (*Adapted from* Lewandowski K, Homenda W, Mital A, et al. Erythrophagocytosis by neutrophils–a rare morphological phenomenon resulting in acquired haemolytic anaemia? Int J Lab Hematol 2011;33(4):448; with permission.)

and is not required if the hemolysis and anemia are mild. Although there are no data to support red cell warmers, they are commonly used if available.

Given that most donor units are P-positive, cross-match-compatible P-positive red cell units are commonly used for transfusion. Only in difficult situations with refractory hemolysis despite supportive measures and transfusion is the rare P-negative blood indicated.[19,26] Antibiotic therapy is effective in putting the chronic hemolysis of syphilis-associated PCH into remission.

Because most cases of acute PCH are transient, they may not require immunosuppressive or pharmacologic drug therapy. Steroids have been tried in patients with severe hemolysis at presentation, but there are no data to show this is beneficial.[20] Plasmapheresis can help mitigate severe acute hemolysis by early clearance of the offending antibody, which can sensitize, detach, and rebind erythrocytes with changes in temperature in the microcirculation.[27]

The anti-CD-20 monoclonal antibody Rituximab has activity in both warm and cold AIHA; there are case reports of Rituximab causing cessation of hemolysis in PCH refractory to other therapies.[28] The recombinant antibody Eculizumab inhibits the terminal part of the complement cascade by binding to C5, inhibiting its cleavage and preventing generation of the terminal membrane attack complex C5b-9. Although intuitively one would expect Eculizumab to effectively inhibit hemolysis in PCH, a single case report was discouraging. The rate of intravascular hemolysis did slow down considerably after Eculizumab was initiated for steroid refractory PCH in an adult patient with multiple myeloma. However, low-grade hemolysis continued possibly from extravascular processes or alternative cell-mediated mechanisms for red cell destruction (such as erythrophagocytosis). The patient ultimately responded to high-dose cyclophosphamide.[29]

SUMMARY

In summary, PCH is rare, but should be recognized early because intervention is simple and effective. Adult hematologists are not very familiar with this entity given its rarity, but should be aware of presentations in association with hematological malignancies. One should work up cases of Coombs-negative immune hemolytic anemia with DL testing. Treatment is predominantly supportive but a variety of immunosuppressive drugs show promise in severe cases.

REFERENCES

1. Sokol RJ, Hewitt S, Stamps BK. Autoimmune haemolysis associated with Donath-Landsteiner antibodies. Acta Haematol 1982;68(4):268–77.
2. Donath JL, Landsteiner K. Uber Paroxysmale Haemoglobinurie. Munch Med Wochenschr 1904;51:1590–3.
3. Jordan WS Jr, Prouty RL, Heinle R, et al. The mechanism of hemolysis in paroxysmal cold hemoglobinuria III. Erythrophagocytosis and leukopenia. Blood 1952; 7(4):387–403.
4. Levine P, Celano MJ, Falkowski F. The specificity of the antibody in paroxysmal cold hemoglobinuria (P.C.H.). Ann N Y Acad Sci 1965;124(2):456–61.
5. Sokol RJ, Hewitt S, Stamps BK, et al. Autoimmune haemolysis in childhood and adolescence. Acta Haematol 1984;72(4):245–57.
6. Vaglio S, Arista MC, Perrone MP, et al. Autoimmune hemolytic anemia in childhood: serologic features in 100 cases. Transfusion 2007;47(1):50–4.
7. Gottsche B, Salama A, Mueller-Eckhardt C. Donath-Landsteiner autoimmune hemolytic anemia in children. A study of 22 cases. Vox Sang 1990;58(4):281–6.
8. Ziman A, Hsi R, Goldfinger D. Transfusion medicine illustrated: Donath-Landsteiner antibody-associated hemolytic anemia after Haemophilus influenzae infection in a child. Transfusion 2004;44(8):1127–8.
9. Bell CA, Zwicker H, Rosenbaum DL. Paroxysmal cold hemoglobinuria (P.C.H.) following mycoplasma infection: anti-I specificity of the biphasic hemolysin. Transfusion 1973;13(3):138–41.
10. Papalia MA, Schwarer AP. Paroxysmal cold haemoglobinuria in an adult with chicken pox. Br J Haematol 2000;109(2):328–9.
11. Colley E. Paroxysmal cold haemoglobin after mumps. Br Med J 1964;1(5397): 1552.
12. Vergara LH, Mota MC, Sarmento Ada G, et al. Acute renal failure secondary to paroxysmal cold hemoglobinuria. An Pediatr (Barc) 2006;64(3):267–9.
13. Hothi DK, Bass P, Morgan M, et al. Acute renal failure in a patient with paroxysmal cold hemoglobinuria. Pediatr Nephrol 2007;22(4):593–6.
14. Mohler DN, Farris BL, Pearre AA. Paroxysmal cold hemoglobinuria with acute renal failure. Arch Intern Med 1963;112(1):36–40.

15. Heddle NM. Acute paroxysmal cold hemoglobinuria. Transfus Med Rev 1989; 3(3):219–29.
16. Mackenzie GM. Paroxysmal hemoglobinuria: a review. Medicine 1929;8(2): 159–92.
17. Sivakumaran M, Murphy PT, Booker DJ, et al. Paroxysmal cold haemoglobinuria caused by non-Hodgkin's lymphoma. Br J Haematol 1999;105(1):278–9.
18. Breccia M, D'Elia GM, Girelli G, et al. Paroxysmal cold haemoglobinuria as a tardive complication of idiopathic myelofibrosis. Eur J Haematol 2004;73(4):304–6.
19. Rausen AR, LeVine R, Hsu TC, et al. Compatible transfusion therapy for paroxysmal cold hemoglobinuria. Pediatrics 1975;55(2):275–8.
20. Wolach B, Heddle N, Barr RD, et al. Transient Donath-Landsteiner haemolytic anaemia. Br J Haematol 1981;48(3):425–34.
21. Depcik-Smith Natalie D, Escobar Miguel A, Ma Alice D, et al. RBC rosetting and erythrophagocytosis in adult paroxysmal cold hemoglobinuria. Transfusion 2001; 41(2):163.
22. Hernandez JA, Steane SM. Erythrophagocytosis by segmented neutrophils in paroxysmal cold hemoglobinuria. Am J Clin Pathol 1984;81(6):787–9.
23. Mukhopadhyay S, Keating L, Souid AK. Erythrophagocytosis in paroxysmal cold hemoglobinuria. Am J Hematol 2003;74(3):196–7.
24. Lewandowski K, Homenda W, Mital A, et al. Erythrophagocytosis by neutrophils– a rare morphological phenomenon resulting in acquired haemolytic anaemia? Int J Lab Hematol 2011;33(4):447–50.
25. Ries CA, Garratty G, Petz LD, et al. Paroxysmal cold hemoglobinuria: report of a case with an exceptionally high thermal range Donath-Landsteiner antibody. Blood 1971;38(4):491–9.
26. Nordhagen R, Stensvold K, Winsnes A, et al. Paroxysmal cold haemoglobinuria. The most frequent acute autoimmune haemolytic anaemia in children? Acta Paediatr Scand 1984;73(2):258–62.
27. Roy-Burman A, Glader BE. Resolution of severe Donath-Landsteiner autoimmune hemolytic anemia temporally associated with institution of plasmapheresis. Crit Care Med 2002;30(4):931–4.
28. Koppel A, Lim S, Osby M, et al. Rituximab as successful therapy in a patient with refractory paroxysmal cold hemoglobinuria. Transfusion 2007;47(10):1902–4.
29. Gregory GP, Opat S, Quach H, et al. Failure of eculizumab to correct paroxysmal cold hemoglobinuria. Ann Hematol 2011;90(8):989–90.

Paroxysmal Nocturnal Hemoglobinuria

A Complement-Mediated Hemolytic Anemia

Amy E. DeZern, MD, MHS[a],*, Robert A. Brodsky, MD[b]

KEYWORDS

- Paroxysmal nocturnal hemoglobinuria • Hemolytic anemia
- Alternative pathway of complement • Humanized anti-C5 monoclonal antibody
- Eculizumab • C3 blockade • C1 inhibition • Bone marrow failure

KEY POINTS

- Paroxysmal nocturnal hemoglobinuria (PNH) is a rare, clonal, hematopoietic stem cell disorder with 3 clinical features: hemolytic anemia from uncontrolled complement activation, thrombosis, and bone marrow failure.
- Eculizumab is a humanized monoclonal antibody that binds to C5 in complement system and decreases intravascular hemolysis, reduces thrombosis risk, and improves quality of life.
- Persistent extravascular hemolysis in PNH while on eculizumab remains a relevant clinical issue and multiple therapies are being examined to improve this.

INTRODUCTION

Paroxysmal nocturnal hemoglobinuria (PNH) is a rare, clonal, hematopoietic stem cell disorder that manifests with a hemolytic anemia from uncontrolled complement activation, bone marrow failure, and a propensity for thrombosis.[1–3] It is the chronic hemolytic anemia in PNH, largely mediated by the alternative pathway of complement (AP), from which the disease derives its descriptive moniker.[2] PNH is a unique disease whose clinical manifestations have been linked to the deficiency in glycosylphosphatidylinositol-anchored proteins (GPI-APs). These manifestations include a lack of the complement regulatory proteins CD55 and CD59.[4] CD55 regulates the formation and stability of the C3 and C5 convertases,[1] whereas CD59 blocks the formation of the membrane attack complex (MAC).[2,5]

[a] Division of Hematologic Malignancies, Department of Oncology, The Bunting and Blaustein Cancer Research Building, 1650 Orleans Street, Room 3M87, Baltimore, MD 21287-0013, USA;
[b] Division of Hematology, The Johns Hopkins University School of Medicine, 720 Rutland Avenue, Ross Research Building, Room 1025, Baltimore, MD 21205, USA
* Corresponding author.
E-mail address: adezern1@jhmi.edu

Hematol Oncol Clin N Am 29 (2015) 479–494
http://dx.doi.org/10.1016/j.hoc.2015.01.005
0889-8588/15/$ – see front matter © 2015 Elsevier Inc. All rights reserved.

The bone marrow failure component of the disease is well-appreciated. The mechanism of the thrombophilia is less well-described. Historically, PNH is among the first diseases in which the role the complement cascade plays in the pathogenesis is well-elucidated. This review focuses on the dysregulation of the complement cascade, leading to the hemolytic anemia in PNH as well as its other clinical manifestations and the therapies available presently and possibly in the future for the disease.

THE PATHOPHYSIOLOGY OF THE COMPLEMENT DYSREGULATION IN PAROXYSMAL NOCTURNAL HEMOGLOBINURIA

The complement system is our host defense system that protects the intravascular space through opsonizing and lysing bacteria. The complement system consists of plasma proteins that interact via 3 major pathways: the classical, alternative, and lectin binding.[6,7] This system encompasses these distinct cascades with individual functions, which all converge into a common final effector mechanism—the MAC (**Fig. 1**). These 3 pathways independently lead to activation of C3 and C5 convertases.[6] Although the classical and the lectin pathways require specific triggers to be activated—usually infection—it has been known for years that the AP exhibits low-grade continuous activation owing to spontaneous hydrolysis of C3 (called the "tick-over" phenomenon).[8–10] In addition, some components of the AP constitute an

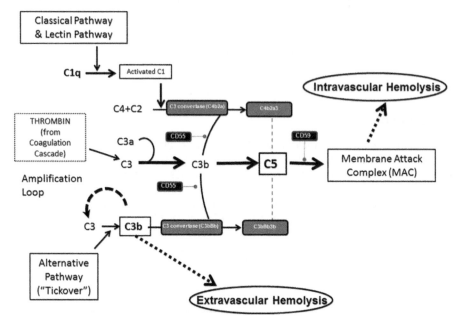

Fig. 1. The complement cascade. The complement cascade is activated via the classical, lectin or alternative pathways. C3 is activated via C3 convertases. This step is regulated by the action of CD55, a glycosylphosphatidylinositol (GPI)-anchored protein. Subsequently, C5 is cleaved into C5a and C5b. C5a mediates a number of biological processes and C5b begins the terminal pathway of complement and the assembly of the membrane attack complex (MAC). The formation of the MAC is regulated by CD59, another GPI-anchored protein. Thrombin interacts with the complement cascade where it can directly cleave C3. Thrombin can also cleave C5 into C5a, which occurs independently of C3 and therefore represents a bypass of the 3 traditional complement activation pathways.

amplification mechanism (the so-called AP amplification loop), which amplifies complement activation regardless of the specific pathway that initially generates the first C3b molecule (see **Fig. 1**). Multiple mechanisms have evolved to control the complement cascade, including membrane-bound proteins (complement receptor 1 [CR1], membrane cofactor protein, and the membrane proteins CD55 and CD59), as well as fluid-phase components, including complement factor I and factor H (FH). Among these, CD55 and CD59 are of pivotal importance in PNH, given that they are normally expressed on hematopoietic cells and attached by the GPI anchor proteins.[11]

With specific respect to the thrombosis seen in PNH, there are many direct and bidirectional interactions between the complement system and the coagulation cascade (see **Fig. 1**, which shows where thrombin interacts). Most notable to the clinical implications is that thrombin can cleave C5 into C5a, which occurs independent of C3 and therefore represents a bypass of the 3 traditional complement activation pathways (that is, the classical, lectin, and APs). Thrombin-activatable fibrinolysis inhibitor inactivates C3a and C5a in a negative feedback loop. The complement system also amplifies coagulation through the C5a-mediated induction of expression of tissue factor and plasminogen activator inhibitor 1 by leukocytes, the latter of which inhibits fibrinolysis.[12] This activation of the complement through the generation of thrombin contributes to hypercoagulability in PNH and may explain why thrombosis in PNH often leads to an inexorable disease flare that is best interrupted by blocking terminal complement.

THE COMPLEMENT PROTEINS IN PAROXYSMAL NOCTURNAL HEMOGLOBINURIA

PNH erythrocytes are highly vulnerable to complement-mediated lysis owing to a reduction, or absence, of 2 important GPI-anchored complement regulatory membrane proteins (CD55 and CD59). CD59 is a glycoprotein that directly prevents the MAC from perforating the cell membrane by blocking the aggregation of C9.[5] CD55 accelerates the rate of destruction of membrane-bound C3 convertase.[13] CD55 (also called decay accelerating factor) inhibits the formation and the stability of C3 convertase (both C3bBb and C4b2a).[14] CD55 was the first complement regulator reported to be absent on PNH erythrocytes.[9,15] CD59 was later identified as an additional complement regulatory protein on PNH erythrocytes.[16] Distinct from CD55, CD59 interferes with the terminal effector complement, blocking the incorporation of C9 onto the C5b–C8 complex, forming the MAC.[17] CD59 is the more important molecule of the two—because, if it is absent, this leads to lysis,[18] whereas an isolated deficiency of CD55 can be overcome. There are patients with a congenital isolated CD55 deficiency but normal CD59 expression who do not hemolyze (see **Fig. 1**).[19]

PAROXYSMAL NOCTURNAL HEMOGLOBINURIA AS A HEMOLYTIC ANEMIA

PNH erythrocytes' in vitro susceptibility to hemolysis was initially described by Dr Ham in his pivotal studies in the 1930s.[20] Dr Ham demonstrated that erythrocytes from patients who have PNH hemolyze in their own serum, especially when the AP is activated (by acidification). This hemolytic assay is called the Ham test or the acidified serum assay.[21] This feature of PNH erythrocytes was subsequently described further when it was demonstrated that a distinct phenotype of PNH erythrocytes may exist, according to their specific sensitivity to complement-mediated lysis in vitro.[22,23] In fact, in PNH there are erythrocytes with only modest hypersensitivity (3–5 times normal values) or a more pronounced hypersensitivity to complement-mediated lysis (15–25 times the normal one). These phenotypes are now known as PNH type II and type III erythrocytes,[23] which by flow cytometry correspond with a complete (type

III) or partial (type II) deficiency of GPI-APs, respectively.[24] Chronic hemolysis of PNH is likely owing to a continuous steady-state complement activation coming from the low-grade spontaneous C3 tick-over, with ongoing activation of the CAP, as described. Infections or inflammatory status usually result in hemolytic crises (the paroxysms that given the disease its name), eventually as a result of substantial complement activation.

PAROXYSMAL NOCTURNAL HEMOGLOBINURIA AS A DISEASE OF MARROW FAILURE

Patient with PNH obviously suffer from anemia, but often they also have other cytopenias in the setting of their marrow failure owing to impaired hematopoiesis. The marrow failure component of PNH can vary from subclinical disease to severe aplastic anemia (AA) and may be categorized as such.[2] It has been demonstrated that PNH patients have a reduced number of hematopoietic progenitors assessed by cultures assays regardless of the categorization.[25,26] There is considerable overlap between PNH and AA both in disease presentation; in addition, they have long been viewed as distinct presentations of the same disorder.[27] The mechanism by which PNH clones expand has been an area of active research. Immunoselection is considered to be essential for the selective expansion of these clones.[28] The expansion is not simply attributable to *PIGA* mutations alone.[29] Also, PNH clonal populations can be detected frequently in patients with the other marrow failure syndromes, such as AA and myelodysplastic syndrome.[30,31] This may suggest that GPI⁻ cells survive immune-mediated bone marrow injury putatively caused by cytotoxic cells such as natural killer cells.[32] Human leukemic K562 cells become relatively resistant to natural killer cell-mediated cytotoxicity after acquisition of *PIGA* mutations in vitro.[33] This relative survival advantage may be owing to deficiency of stress-inducible GPI-linked membrane proteins upregulation of UL16-binding protein (ULBP)1 and ULBP2 on PNH cells. ULBPs activate natural killer and T cells and are detected on GPI-expressing but not on GPI-deficient K562 cells. Thus, in the setting of an immune attack on the bone marrow, the lack of ULBPs may contribute to immunoselection of the PNH clone over normal cells.[34] There also is the view that the patients with PNH clones and the autoimmune phenomenon of AA have an attack against the hematopoiesis at the level of the stem cell, and this allows the clonal expansion for the clinical PNH phenotype.[35] More recently, it has been suggested that the GPI-AP could be the target of the immune attack and thus the PNH cells are spared naturally, again allowing their clonal outgrowth over the normal hematopoiesis.[36] The PNH clone is often considered a marker of an immune form of marrow failure because it may predict response to immunosuppressive therapy in AA and patients with inherited forms of AA lack the PNH clone.[37] The size of the PNH clone may vary over time and this is the best determinant of the hemolytic component of the disease.[38–41] Therapies directed at this hemolysis will not improve the patients' marrow failure.

PAROXYSMAL NOCTURNAL HEMOGLOBINURIA AS A DISEASE OF THROMBOSIS

Thrombosis is another typical manifestation of PNH. It is the leading cause of death in the disease.[42] Thrombosis may occur at any site in PNH: venous or arterial. Common sites include intraabdominal (hepatic, portal, splenic or mesenteric) and cerebral (cavernous or sagittal sinus) veins, with hepatic vein thrombosis (also known as Budd–Chiari syndrome) being the most common. Deep venous thrombosis, pulmonary emboli, and dermal thrombosis are also prevalent. In contrast with the mechanisms of the hemolysis or the marrow failure, less is definitively known about the pathophysiology and mechanism of the thrombophilia in PNH, especially in patients not treated with eculizumab. Clinically, the complication of thrombosis is more prevalent in patients as the PNH clone increases in size.[42–44] Thrombosis may occur in any PNH patient, but those with a large percentage of PNH cells (>50% granulocytes) are at greatest risk.[44,45] This may suggest that the ultimate etiology of the thrombophilia in PNH is related to the hemolysis with complement activation. As discussed, there are also clear interactions between the complement system and the coagulation cascade, namely thrombin and C3, which contribute to the thrombosis in PNH. There are currently several hypothesized mechanisms and ultimately the pathophysiology may be multifactorial. The thrombophilia may directly result from the hemolytic anemia as the free hemoglobin is released by the erythrocytes into the serum causing nitric oxide (NO) scavenging and thus preventing the inhibition by NO on platelet aggregation and adhesion to endothelium.[46] Next, the uncontrolled complement regulation on platelet surface could be hypothesized to lead to platelet activation and aggregation, enhancing the formation of thrombi.[47] Another known issue is that the absence of GPI-APs on PNH platelets leads to thrombotic microparticles.[48] Another possible mechanism of thrombosis in PNH could be a disruption of the fibrinolytic system, owing to the lack of membrane-bound urokinase-type plasminogen activator receptor, another GPI-anchored protein, leaving excess of its soluble form.[49,50] Complement activation also contributes to the prothrombotic tendency of PNH patients. Specifically, C5a may result in proinflammatory and prothrombotic processes by generating inflammatory cytokines such as interleukin-6, interleukin-8, and tumor necrosis factor.[51] It is unclear which of these mechanisms contribute most to thrombosis in PNH; however, complement inhibition with eculizumab is the most effective means to stop thrombosis in PNH.[52,53] Anticoagulation and eculizumab are indication for acute thrombotic events; however, primary prophylactic anticoagulation has not been proven to be beneficial in PNH.[42] Anticoagulation after the acute event in a PNH patient well-maintained on eculizumab may not be necessary.[54]

PAROXYSMAL NOCTURNAL HEMOGLOBINURIA AND CONSEQUENCES OF NITRIC OXIDE

Many manifestations of PNH result from intravascular hemolysis and are explained by hemoglobin-mediated NO scavenging after free hemoglobin is released from hemolyzed cells.[46] NO is a major regulator of vascular physiology. NO acts on the vascular wall to maintain normal tone and limit platelet activation. Free hemoglobin has enormous affinity for NO and can reduce the plasma level of NO to the point of causing symptoms. This reduction has been demonstrated in clinical trials where the administration of cell-free hemoglobin solutions to healthy people is associated with development of abdominal pain and esophageal spasm.[55] Under normal conditions, hemoglobin is sequestered by the erythrocyte membrane, which minimizes the scavenging of NO. In PNH, the intravascular hemolysis results in release of large amounts of free hemoglobin into the plasma. This release leads to scavenging of NO and degradation of the substrate for NO synthesis.[56,57] This depletion of NO at the tissue level manifests clinically as fatigue, abdominal pain, esophageal spasm, erectile dysfunction, and possibly thrombosis. These clinical symptoms are more common in patients with PNH who have larger populations of PNH cells (>60% of granulocytes).[44] Additionally, chronic kidney disease and pulmonary hypertension are complications that may go unrecognized, but also result from scavenging of NO. For example, in pulmonary arterial hypertension the symptoms are usually mild and are often nonspecific (eg, tiredness, breathlessness). Chronic kidney disease stages 1 through 3 are also described and can be quite common in PNH patients.[58]

DIAGNOSIS AND CLASSIFICATION OF PAROXYSMAL NOCTURNAL HEMOGLOBINURIA

The diagnosis of PNH is both a laboratory and a clinical diagnosis. The laboratory measures include a reticulocyte count, lactate dehydrogenase (LDH) levels, complete blood count indicative of hemolysis, and peripheral blood flow cytometry to detect the deficiency of the GPI (**Box 1**).[59] This absence of GPI-APs is detected after staining cells with monoclonal antibodies and a reagent known as fluorescein-tagged proaerolysin variant that binds the glycan portion of the GPI anchor.[60] The erythrocytes may be classified as types I, II, or III PNH cells, as noted. Type I cells have normal levels of CD55 and CD59, whereas type II have reduced levels and type III have complete absence.[2] Hematopathologists have recently published guidelines for diagnosis of PNH using flow cytometry.[61]

The classification of PNH has been proposed by the International PNH Interest Group (IPIG)[2] and includes 3 subtypes: classical PNH, which includes hemolytic and thrombotic patients who have evidence of PNH in the absence of another bone marrow failure disorder; PNH in the context of other primary bone marrow disorders, such as AA or myelodysplastic syndrome; and subclinical PNH, in which patients have small PNH clones but no clinical or laboratory evidence of hemolysis or thrombosis.[2]

Box 1
Clinical care of PNH patients

Diagnosis
- PNH by FLAER assay
- LDH
- Reticulocyte count
- CBC

Therapy
- Eculizumab intravenously
  - Loading: 600 mg weekly × 4 weeks
  - Maintenance (followed 1 week later): 900 mg every 2 weeks thereafter
- Consideration of HSCT in suboptimal responders

Monitoring while on therapy
- At least monthly
  - LDH, reticulocyte count, CBC, chemistries
- At least yearly
  - PNH by FLAER assay
- If concern for extravascular hemolysis
  - Direct antiglobulin test

Abbreviations: CBC, complete blood count; FLAER, fluorescein-tagged proaerolysin variant; HSCT, hematopoietic stem cell transplantation; LDH, lactate dehydrogenase; PNH, paroxysmal nocturnal hemoglobinuria.
Laboratory testing for diagnosis and monitoring during treatment. Standard therapy regimen with eculizumab.

CURRENT THERAPIES FOR PAROXYSMAL NOCTURNAL HEMOGLOBINURIA DIRECTED AGAINST COMPLEMENT

Eculizumab is a humanized monoclonal antibody that binds to C5 and inhibits its further cleavage into C5a and C5b. The drug decreases intravascular hemolysis, reduces thrombosis risk, and improves quality of life in PNH[52,62] by inhibiting the formation of the MAC (**Fig. 2**).[63] It is the only therapy approved by the US Food and Drug Administration for PNH.

Eculizumab was studied originally in a pilot trial published in the *New England Journal of Medicine*, which showed that it was safe and well-tolerated in PNH patients. This pilot study demonstrated also that LDH levels in these patients with transfusion-dependent anemia from their PNH decreased as intravascular hemolysis was blocked with the drug.[64] These principles were demonstrated further in a larger, multicenter, randomized, placebo-controlled, blinded study in 86 PNH patients. Eculizumab was administered intravenously at 600 mg weekly for 4 weeks, followed 1 week later by 900 mg every 2 weeks thereafter (see **Box 1**).[65] Again, therapy with eculizumab

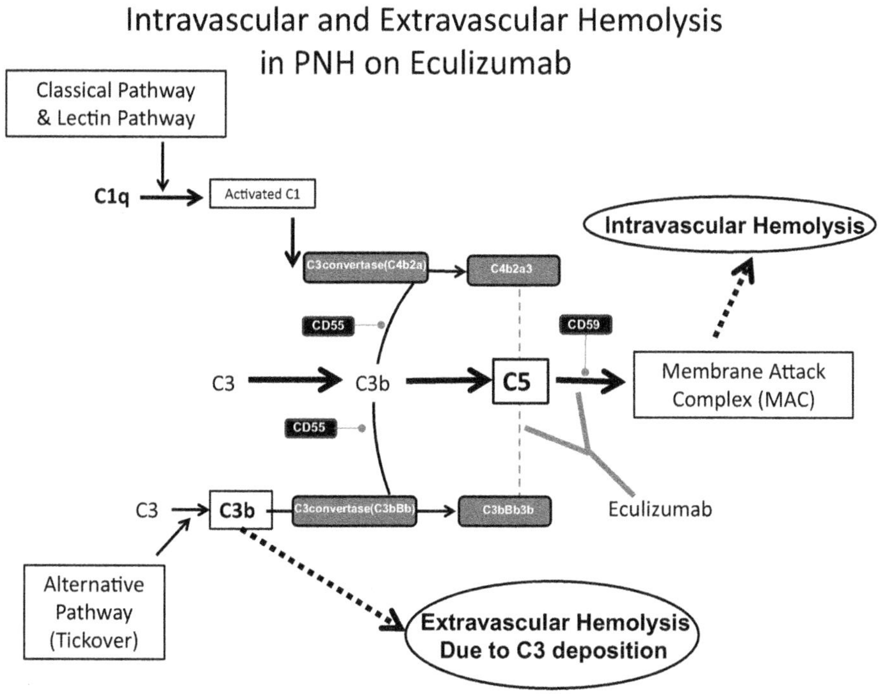

Fig. 2. The complement cascade, paroxysmal nocturnal hemoglobinuria (PNH), and eculizumab. PNH cells have a deficiency in glycosylphosphatidylinositol-anchored proteins on their cell surface. Absence of CD55 and CD59 leads to uncontrolled complement activation on the surface of PNH cells. Deficiency of CD59 increases MAC formation and induces intravascular hemolysis, which is central to the pathophysiology of PNH. Deficiency of CD55 leads to increased C3 convertase activity and C3d-associated extravascular hemolysis. Eculizumab therapy for PNH is a humanized monoclonal antibody that targets C5. By preventing C5 activation, eculizumab prevents the formation of the MAC, leading to a significant reduction in intravascular hemolysis of PNH cells. Use of eculizumab can lead to increased extravascular hemolysis.

resulted decreased intravascular hemolysis, as measured by LDH, and transfusion independence in about one-half of the patients. There was also the disappearance of many of the clinical symptoms of intravascular hemolysis, including fatigue, esophageal spasm, and erectile dysfunction in the PNH patients on eculizumab arm in comparison with placebo. This second study again proved that eculizumab treatment was safe with few adverse events, even in comparison with the placebo. A third study of eculizumab (open-label phase III study SHEPHERD[62]) was conducted with broader inclusion criteria for the PNH patients, allowing for minimally transfused patients as well as those with more pronounced thrombocytopenia. In the 96 patients enrolled in the study, treatment with eculizumab resulted again in intravascular hemolysis, regardless of the severity of disease before therapy. Transfusion independence was achieved in about one-half of the patients and improvement in fatigue and quality of life were demonstrated as well.[62] The study of eculizumab continued in the final open-label extension study. This extension included 187 patients who have previously been treated on the parent clinical trials.[52] The extension study confirmed the safety and efficacy of eculizumab as well. More recently, additional follow-up data has been published, again with same findings.[66]

Patients require close monitoring while on eculizumab treatment (see **Box 1**). Standardly, peripheral blood work should include a reticulocyte count, LDH, complete blood count, and chemistries (including bilirubin) weekly during induction therapy. Thereafter, the same laboratory tests should be checked every 4 weeks. Also a direct antiglobulin test (Coombs' test) should be obtained in patients with evidence of persistent hemolysis while on therapy. This may alert the clinician to ongoing extravascular hemolysis that the eculizumab and its downstream C3 deposition are causing. PNH flow cytometry should be obtained at least every 6 to 12 months because the clone size may vary over time. The measure of hemolysis (LDH) in a therapy responder usually fall within the normal range within days to weeks after starting eculizumab; however, the reticulocyte count usually remains elevated and the hemoglobin response can vary by patient and time.

PREDICTORS OF RESPONSE TO ECULIZUMAB THERAPY

The majority of classical PNH patients respond to eculizumab; however, the hemoglobin response is highly variable and may depend on underlying bone marrow failure, concurrent inflammatory conditions, genetic factors, and the size of the PNH red cell clone after therapy.[39] However, there are limitations to this therapy and not all patients have their disease-specific needs met by eculizumab.[39] There have been observed clinical scenarios that seem to predict for either breakthrough hemolysis or a poor response to eculizumab. As previously reported, eculizumab does not improve underlying bone marrow failure.[67] There are also reports of patients who have a coexistent autoimmune disease (2 with Crohn's disease, 1 with Graves' disease, and 1 with rheumatoid arthritis) with ongoing activation of complement from their underlying disease, which lead to suboptimal responses from eculizumab.[39] Breakthrough hemolysis is a challenge in these patients. Although the mechanism for this potential association is unclear, it is conceivable that chronic inflammatory states lead to increased complement activation that requires high dosages of eculizumab because standard doses resulted in incomplete C5 blockade. It is also known that transient breakthrough intravascular hemolysis is observed after viral or bacterial infections.[39]

Another group of suboptimal responders to eculizumab has been described recently. A single missense C5 heterozygous mutation, c.2654G → A, prevents binding and blockade by eculizumab while retaining the functional capacity to cause hemolysis. The polymorphism accounts for the poor response to eculizumab in patients carrying the mutation. The c.2654G→A mutation is present in 3.5% of the Japanese population and has not yet been described in other ethnic groups.[68] Pharmacogenetics has also been shown to influence response to therapy. Polymorphisms in the CR1 gene are associated with response to eculizumab. CR1, through binding C3b and C4b, enhances the decay of the C3 and C5 convertases. The density of CR1 on the surface of red cells modulates binding of C3 fragments to the GPI-negative red cells when C5 is inhibited. PNH patients with polymorphisms in CR1 that lead to low CR1 levels (L/L genotype) are more likely to be suboptimal responders to eculizumab than patients with intermediate (H/L genotype) or high (H/H genotype) levels of CR1.[69]

Pregnancy can be another limitation on the efficacy of eculizumab. Pregnancy is a hypercoagulable state itself and there have been concerns both about the potential for increased maternal and fetal morbidity in a pregnant patient as well as the safety of eculizumab therapy in pregnancy. There are multiple case reports in the literature of successful pregnancies in female patients on eculizumab.[70–73] However, what has been shown is that these pregnant patients tend to experience increased breakthrough hemolysis as they progress through the trimesters and often require reduced dosing interval (to 12 or even 7 days between doses) by the third trimester. This may be owing to increased activation of the complement cascade with increase terminal complex formation in the third trimester of pregnancy and/or increased volume of distribution of the drug during the latter stage of pregnancy.[73]

CURE FOR PAROXYSMAL NOCTURNAL HEMOGLOBINURIA: HEMATOPOIETIC STEM CELL TRANSPLANTATION

Hematopoietic stem cell transplantation (HSCT) is the only curative therapy for PNH. However, it is not recommended as initial therapy in the eculizumab era, given the risks of transplant-related morbidity and mortality. HSCT is a reasonable therapeutic option in patients who do not respond to therapy with eculizumab[39,74] or those patients who have severe pancytopenia owing to underlying bone marrow failure. The transplant paradigm pursued is often with reduced intensity conditioning regimens, because myeloablation is not required to eradicate the PNH clone.[75] The use of HSCT may be studied more in the future as patients and their health care providers determine that the cost–benefit ratio of HSCT outweighs a lifetime of eculizumab therapy.

FUTURE THERAPIES FOR PAROXYSMAL NOCTURNAL HEMOGLOBINURIA DIRECTED AGAINST COMPLEMENT

There continue to be challenges in therapies for PNH patients, both when eculizumab results in suboptimal response as well as with new drugs. The reasons for this are 2-fold. One is that, by blocking the terminal pathway of complement, an arm of immunity is simultaneously blocked, which prevents the formation of the MAC, which is needed to protect against infections, especially *Neisseria*. Therefore, patients who are on eculizumab therapy are usually more susceptible to infections caused by meningococcus or gonococcus. However, this can be overcome by way of a vaccine against meningococci or prophylactic antibiotics such as a fluroquinolone. The other challenge is that the therapy only influences a certain part of complement activities. It allows the immunoprotection and immunoregulation functions mediated by C3b to be retained. This function can be beneficial for patients, because it allows them to maintain their immune defense.[58] Eculizumab compensates for the CD59 deficiency on PNH erythrocytes, but not the CD55 deficiency. Thus, PNH patients on eculizumab accumulate C3 fragments on their CD55-deficient red cells, leading to extravascular hemolysis through the accumulation of opsonins that are recognized by the reticulo-endothelial system (see **Fig. 2**).[76] Laboratory evidence of extravascular hemolysis in eculizumab-containing patients includes increased reticulocytes, persistent anemia, and often direct antiglobulin testing that is positive for C3 deposition. These patients may remain asymptomatic, but others have symptomatic anemia and remain dependent on transfusions.[39] Thus, there is need for additional work toward a complement inhibitor that reduces C3 accumulation on PNH erythrocytes.

The evidence that C3 activation represents a potential target, unique from C5 blockade, for complement modulation is an ongoing area of research both in vitro and in vivo. However, there have been concerns that C3 inhibitor might be associated with increased infectious toxicity.[77] Nonetheless, active research is ongoing to study this therapeutic possibility.

There is an antibody-based anti-C3 strategy that targets activated C3 (C3b/iC3b). This anti-C3b/iC3b murine monoclonal antibody 3E7 and its chimeric-deimmunized derivative H17 were shown to selectively inhibit the activity of C3 and C5 convertases of the CAP only, providing the opportunity for a selective inhibition of different complement pathway.[78] These antibodies were tested in vitro on PNH erythrocytes, and were shown to be effective in preventing complement-mediated hemolysis of CD55/CD59 deficient erythrocytes.[78] This approach has yet to be translated into the clinic.

Targeted C3 complement inhibition has also included strategies based on small peptide inhibitors, which may be closer to clinical translation. The best example of this is compstatin, which selectively binds to C3 and its active fragment C3b.[79,80] Compstatin prevents the conversion of C3 to C3b and thus it impairs all initiation, amplification, and terminal pathways of the complement cascade.[81] Preliminary data show that compstatin analogs inhibit complement activation on PNH erythrocytes, preventing both hemolysis and C3 deposition.[82] There are also ongoing investigations of peptidic C3 inhibitor, compstatin Cp40, and its long-acting form (polyethylene glycol–Cp40) in PNH in vitro models. Thus, peptide inhibitors of C3 activation effectively prevent hemolysis and C3 opsonization of PNH erythrocytes[83] and are another potential therapeutic in this disease.

A similar but distinct path that could also inhibit complement in these PNH patients involves C1 esterase inhibitor (C1INH). This is an endogenous human plasma protein in the family of serine protease inhibitors (SERPINs) and it has broad inhibitory activity in the complement and coagulation pathways. C1INH inhibits the classical pathway of complement by binding C1r and C1s and inhibits the mannose-binding, lectin-associated serine proteases in the lectin pathway.[84,85] It has already been shown in humans that the commercially available plasma derived C1INH (Cinryze) prevents PNH erythrocyte lysis induced by the AP.[86] Importantly, C1INH was able to block the accumulation of C3 degradation products on CD55-deficient erythrocytes from PNH patients on therapy with eculizumab in vitro.[86] This is significant clinically in patients treated with eculizumab who fail to achieve transfusion independence.[39,66,87] Patients who do not respond to eculizumab therapy could theoretically respond to a C1INH, either alone or in combination with C5 blockade. A clinical trial is anticipated to explore this hypothesis in vivo.

Last, strategies of complement inhibition that deliver a selective inhibition of early phases (C3 activation) of the AP of the complement cascade are being developed. These strategies retain intact functioning of the other 2 complement pathways. This strategy uses FH, a complement inhibitor that modulates the initial AP activation in the fluid phase by preventing C3 convertase activity and by promoting C3b inactivation into iC3b.[88] FH modulates the AP amplification loop and it has been demonstrated to inhibit lysis in vitro.[89] There are 2 FH-derived agents currently studied. The first is TT30, which is a recombinant fusion protein between complement FH and another complement-related protein, complement receptor 2, which delivers FH activity locally at the site of complement activation. This was investigated in an in vitro model, which showed that TT30 completely inhibited complement-mediated hemolysis of PNH erythrocytes and effectively prevents initial C3 activation and further C3 deposition on PNH erythrocytes.[90] There was a phase I clinical trial for PNH patients to study the use of TT30 (clinicaltrials.gov) that was closed owing to inability to enroll. Mini-FH is the second analogous agent that results in selective inhibition of activation and amplification of the AP, without affecting the other 2 pathways. Mini-FH was found to be more effective than TT30, with full inhibition achieved at concentrations about 1 log lower than TT30.[91] This has yet to be translated into the clinic to date.

SUMMARY

PNH is caused by a somatic mutation in *PIGA* that leads to a marked deficiency or absence of the complement regulatory proteins CD55 and CD59. The disease manifests with intravascular hemolysis, bone marrow failure, and thrombosis. Complement inhibition through the C5 monoclonal antibody eculizumab has led to dramatic clinical improvement in PNH. Although this therapeutic approach is safe and effective, there is residual complement activity resulting from upstream complement components that account for suboptimal responses in patients. A novel era for complement regulation in PNH is upon us and the goal is to find targeted and specific treatments for PNH and other complement-mediated diseases.

REFERENCES

1. Rosse WF. Paroxysmal nocturnal hemoglobinuria as a molecular disease. Medicine 1997;76(2):63–93.
2. Parker C, Omine M, Richards S, et al. Diagnosis and management of paroxysmal nocturnal hemoglobinuria. Blood 2005;106(12):3699–709.
3. Brodsky RA. Narrative review: paroxysmal nocturnal hemoglobinuria: the physiology of complement-related hemolytic anemia. Ann Intern Med 2008;148(8): 587–95.
4. Miyata T, Yamada N, Iida Y, et al. Abnormalities of PIG-A transcripts in granulocytes from patients with paroxysmal nocturnal hemoglobinuria. N Engl J Med 1994;330:249–55.
5. Rollins SA, Sims PJ. The complement-inhibitory activity of CD59 resides in its capacity to block incorporation of C9 into membrane C5b-9. J Immunol 1990; 144(9):3478–83.
6. Walport MJ. Complement. First of two parts. N Engl J Med 2001;344(14): 1058–66.
7. Walport MJ. Complement. Second of two parts. N Engl J Med 2001;344(15): 1140–4.
8. Holt DS, Botto M, Bygrave AE, et al. Targeted deletion of the CD59 gene causes spontaneous intravascular hemolysis and hemoglobinuria. Blood 2001;98(2): 442–9.
9. Pangburn MK, Schreiber RD, Muller-Eberhard HJ. Deficiency of an erythrocyte membrane protein with complement regulatory activity in paroxysmal nocturnal hemoglobinuria. Proc Natl Acad Sci U S A 1983;80(17):5430–4.

10. Pangburn MK, Muller-Eberhard HJ. Initiation of the alternative complement pathway due to spontaneous hydrolysis of the thioester of C3. Ann N Y Acad Sci 1983;421:291–8.
11. Medof ME, Gottlieb A, Kinoshita T, et al. Relationship between decay accelerating factor deficiency, diminished acetylcholinesterase activity, and defective terminal complement pathway restriction in paroxysmal nocturnal hemoglobinuria erythrocytes. J Clin Invest 1987;80(1):165–74.
12. Rittirsch D, Flierl MA, Ward PA. Harmful molecular mechanisms in sepsis. Nat Rev Immunol 2008;8(10):776–87.
13. Medof ME, Kinoshita T, Nussenzweig V. Inhibition of complement activation on the surface of cells after incorporation of decay-accelerating factor (DAF) into their membranes. J Exp Med 1984;160:1558–78.
14. Nicholson-Weller A, March JP, Rosenfeld SI, et al. Affected erythrocytes of patients with paroxysmal nocturnal hemoglobinuria are deficient in the complement regulatory protein, decay accelerating factor. Proc Natl Acad Sci U S A 1983; 80(16):5066–70.
15. Pangburn MK, Schreiber RD, Muller-Eberhard HJ. C3b deposition during activation of the alternative complement pathway and the effect of deposition on the activating surface. J Immunol 1983;131(4):1930–5.
16. Holguin MH, Fredrick LR, Bernshaw NJ, et al. Isolation and characterization of a membrane protein from normal human erythrocytes that inhibits reactive lysis of the erythrocytes of paroxysmal nocturnal hemoglobinuria. J Clin Invest 1989; 84(1):7–17.
17. Meri S, Morgan BP, Davies A, et al. Human protectin (CD59), an 18,000–20,000 MW complement lysis restricting factor, inhibits C5b-8 catalysed insertion of C9 into lipid bilayers. Immunology 1990;71(1):1–9.
18. Wilcox LA, Ezzell JL, Bernshaw NJ, et al. Molecular basis of the enhanced susceptibility of the erythrocytes of paroxysmal nocturnal hemoglobinuria to hemolysis in acidified serum. Blood 1991;78(3):820–9.
19. Telen MJ, Green AM. The Inab phenotype: characterization of the membrane protein and complement regulatory defect. Blood 1989;74(1):437–41.
20. Ham TH. Chronic hemolytic anemia with paroxysmal nocturnal hemoglobinuria. A study of the mechanism of hemolysisin relation to acid-base equilibrium. N Engl J Med 1937;217:915–7.
21. Ham TH, Dingle JH. Studies on destruction of red blood cells. II. Chronic hemolytic anemia with paroxysmal nocturnal hemoglobinuria: certain immunological aspects of the hemolytic mechanism with special reference to serum complement. J Clin Invest 1939;18(6):657–72.
22. Rosse WF, Dacie JV. Immune lysis of normal human and paroxysmal nocturnal hemoglobinuria (PNH) red blood cells. I. The sensitivity of PNH red cells to lysis by complement and specific antibody. J Clin Invest 1966; 45(5):736–48.
23. Rosse WF. The life-span of complement-sensitive and -insensitive red cells in paroxysmal nocturnal hemoglobinuria. Blood 1971;37(5):556–62.
24. Vanderschoot CE, Huizinga TW, van 't Veer-Korthof ET, et al. Deficiency of glycosyl-phosphatidylinositol-linked membrane glycoproteins of leukocytes in paroxysmal nocturnal hemoglobinuria, description of a new diagnostic cytoflourometric assay. Blood 1990;76(9):1853–9.
25. Rotoli B, Robledo R, Scarpato N, et al. Two populations of erythroid cell progenitors in paroxysmal nocturnal hemoglobinuria. Blood 1984;64(4): 847–51.

26. Maciejewski JP, Sloand EM, Sato T, et al. Impaired hematopoiesis in paroxysmal nocturnal hemoglobinuria/aplastic anemia is not associated with a selective proliferative defect in the glycosylphosphatidylinositol-anchored protein-deficient clone. Blood 1997;89(4):1173–81.
27. Dameshek W. Riddle: what do aplastic anemia, paroxysmal nocturnal hemoglobinuria (PNH) and "hypoplastic" leukemia have in common? (Editorial). Blood 1967;30(2):251–4.
28. Nakakuma H, Kawaguchi T. Pathogenesis of selective expansion of PNH clones. Int J Hematol 2003;77(2):121–4.
29. Inoue N, Izui-Sarumaru T, Murakami Y, et al. Molecular basis of clonal expansion of hematopoiesis in 2 patients with paroxysmal nocturnal hemoglobinuria (PNH). Blood 2006;108(13):4232–6.
30. Iwanaga M, Furukawa K, Amenomori T, et al. Paroxysmal nocturnal haemoglobinuria clones in patients with myelodysplastic syndromes. Br J Haematol 1998; 102(2):465–74.
31. Griscelli-Bennaceur A, Gluckman E, Scrobohaci ML, et al. Aplastic anemia and paroxysmal nocturnal hemoglobinuria: search for a pathogenetic link. Blood 1995;85:1354–63.
32. Bessler M, Mason P, Hillmen P, et al. Somatic mutations and cellular selection in paroxysmal nocturnal haemoglobinuria. Lancet 1994;343(8903):951–3.
33. Nagakura S, Ishihara S, Dunn DE, et al. Decreased susceptibility of leukemic cells with PIG-A mutation to natural killer cells in vitro. Blood 2002;100(3): 1031–7.
34. Hanaoka N, Kawaguchi T, Horikawa K, et al. Immunoselection by natural killer cells of PIGA mutant cells missing stress-inducible ULBP. Blood 2006;107(3): 1184–91.
35. Lewis SM, Dacie JV. The aplastic anaemia–paroxysmal nocturnal haemoglobinuria syndrome. Br J Haematol 1967;13(2):236–51.
36. Gargiulo L, Papaioannou M, Sica M, et al. Glycosylphosphatidylinositol-specific, CD1d-restricted T cells in paroxysmal nocturnal hemoglobinuria. Blood 2013; 121(14):2753–61.
37. Dezern AE, Symons HJ, Resar LS, et al. Detection of paroxysmal nocturnal hemoglobinuria clones to exclude inherited bone marrow failure syndromes. Eur J Haematol 2014;92:467–70.
38. Scheinberg P, Marte M, Nunez O, et al. Paroxysmal nocturnal hemoglobinuria clones in severe aplastic anemia patients treated with horse anti-thymocyte globulin plus cyclosporine. Haematologica 2010;95(7):1075–80.
39. DeZern AE, Dorr D, Brodsky RA. Predictors of hemoglobin response to eculizumab therapy in paroxysmal nocturnal hemoglobinuria. Eur J Haematol 2013; 90(1):16–24.
40. Sugimori C, Chuhjo T, Feng X, et al. Minor population of CD55-CD59- blood cells predicts response to immunosuppressive therapy and prognosis in patients with aplastic anemia. Blood 2006;107(4):1308–14.
41. Nakao S, Sugimori C, Yamazaki H. Clinical significance of a small population of paroxysmal nocturnal hemoglobinuria-type cells in the management of bone marrow failure. Int J Hematol 2006;84(2):118–22.
42. Hill A, Kelly RJ, Hillmen P. Thrombosis in paroxysmal nocturnal hemoglobinuria. Blood 2013;121(25):4985–96 [quiz: 5105].
43. Hall C, Richards S, Hillmen P. Primary prophylaxis with warfarin prevents thrombosis in paroxysmal nocturnal hemoglobinuria (PNH). Blood 2003;102(10): 3587–91.

44. Moyo VM, Mukhina GL, Garrett ES, et al. Natural history of paroxysmal nocturnal hemoglobinuria using modern diagnostic assays. Br J Haematol 2004;126:133–8.

45. Nishimura J, Kanakura Y, Ware RE, et al. Clinical course and flow cytometric analysis of paroxysmal nocturnal hemoglobinuria in the United States and Japan. Medicine (Baltimore) 2004;83(3):193–207.

46. Rother RP, Bell L, Hillmen P, et al. The clinical sequelae of intravascular hemolysis and extracellular plasma hemoglobin: a novel mechanism of human disease. JAMA 2005;293(13):1653–62.

47. Louwes H, Vellenga E, de Wolf JT. Abnormal platelet adhesion on abdominal vessels in asymptomatic patients with paroxysmal nocturnal hemoglobinuria. Ann Hematol 2001;80(10):573–6.

48. Wiedmer T, Hall SE, Ortel TL, et al. Complement-induced vesiculation and exposure of membrane prothrombinase sites in platelets of paroxysmal nocturnal hemoglobinuria. Blood 1993;82(4):1192–6.

49. Ninomiya H, Hasegawa Y, Nagasawa T, et al. Excess soluble urokinase-type plasminogen activator receptor in the plasma of patients with paroxysmal nocturnal hemoglobinuria inhibits cell-associated fibrinolytic activity. Int J Hematol 1997;65(3):285–91.

50. Sloand EM, Pfannes L, Scheinberg P, et al. Increased soluble urokinase plasminogen activator receptor (suPAR) is associated with thrombosis and inhibition of plasmin generation in paroxysmal nocturnal hemoglobinuria (PNH) patients. Exp Hematol 2008;36(12):1616–24.

51. Ritis K, Doumas M, Mastellos D, et al. A novel C5a receptor-tissue factor crosstalk in neutrophils links innate immunity to coagulation pathways. J Immunol 2006;177(7):4794–802.

52. Hillmen P, Muus P, Dührsen U, et al. Effect of the complement inhibitor eculizumab on thromboembolism in patients with paroxysmal nocturnal hemoglobinuria. Blood 2007;110(12):4123–8.

53. Weitz IC, Razavi P, Rochanda L, et al. Eculizumab therapy results in rapid and sustained decreases in markers of thrombin generation and inflammation in patients with PNH independent of its effects on hemolysis and microparticle formation. Thromb Res 2012;130(3):361–8.

54. Emadi A, Brodsky RA. Successful discontinuation of anticoagulation following eculizumab administration in paroxysmal nocturnal hemoglobinuria. Am J Hematol 2009;84(10):699–701.

55. Carmichael FJ. Recent developments in hemoglobin-based oxygen carriers–an update on clinical trials. Transfus Apher Sci 2001;24(1):17–21.

56. Azizi E, Dror Y, Wallis K. Arginase activity in erythrocytes of healthy and ill children. Clin Chim Acta 1970;28(3):391–6.

57. Morris CR, Kato GJ, Poljakovic M, et al. Dysregulated arginine metabolism, hemolysis-associated pulmonary hypertension, and mortality in sickle cell disease. JAMA 2005;294(1):81–90.

58. Heitlinger E. Learnings from over 25 years of PNH experience: the era of targeted complement inhibition. Blood Rev 2013;27(Suppl 1):S1–6.

59. Brodsky RA. How I treat paroxysmal nocturnal hemoglobinuria. Blood 2009; 113(26):6522–7.

60. Brodsky RA, Mukhina GL, Li S, et al. Improved detection and characterization of paroxysmal nocturnal hemoglobinuria using fluorescent aerolysin. Am J Clin Pathol 2000;114(3):459–66.

61. Borowitz MJ, Craig FE, Digiuseppe JA, et al. Guidelines for the diagnosis and monitoring of paroxysmal nocturnal hemoglobinuria and related disorders by flow cytometry. Cytometry B Clin Cytom 2010;78(4):211–30.

62. Brodsky RA, Young NS, Antonioli E, et al. Multicenter phase 3 study of the complement inhibitor eculizumab for the treatment of patients with paroxysmal nocturnal hemoglobinuria. Blood 2008;111(4):1840–7.
63. Rother RP, Rollins SA, Mojcik CF, et al. Discovery and development of the complement inhibitor eculizumab for the treatment of paroxysmal nocturnal hemoglobinuria. Nat Biotechnol 2007;25(11):1256–64.
64. Hillmen P, Hall C, Marsh JC, et al. Effect of eculizumab on hemolysis and transfusion requirements in patients with paroxysmal nocturnal hemoglobinuria. N Engl J Med 2004;350(6):552–9.
65. Hillmen P, Young NS, Schubert J, et al. The complement inhibitor eculizumab in paroxysmal nocturnal hemoglobinuria. N Engl J Med 2006;355(12):1233–43.
66. Hillmen P, Muus P, Röth A, et al. Long-term safety and efficacy of sustained eculizumab treatment in patients with paroxysmal nocturnal haemoglobinuria. Br J Haematol 2013;162:62–73.
67. Kelly RJ, Hill A, Arnold LM, et al. Long-term treatment with eculizumab in paroxysmal nocturnal hemoglobinuria: sustained efficacy and improved survival. Blood 2011;117(25):6786–92.
68. Nishimura J, Yamamoto M, Hayashi S, et al. Genetic variants in C5 and poor response to eculizumab. N Engl J Med 2014;370(7):632–9.
69. Rondelli T, Risitano AM, Peffault de Latour R, et al. Polymorphism of the complement receptor 1 gene correlates with the hematologic response to eculizumab in patients with paroxysmal nocturnal hemoglobinuria. Haematologica 2014;99(2): 262–6.
70. Kelly R, Arnold L, Richards S, et al. The management of pregnancy in paroxysmal nocturnal haemoglobinuria on long term eculizumab. Br J Haematol 2010;149(3): 446–50.
71. Marasca R, Coluccio V, Santachiara R, et al. Pregnancy in PNH: another eculizumab baby. Br J Haematol 2010;150(6):707–8.
72. Danilov AV, Brodsky RA, Craigo S, et al. Managing a pregnant patient with paroxysmal nocturnal hemoglobinuria in the era of eculizumab. Leuk Res 2010;34(5): 566–71.
73. Townsley DM, Young NS. Blood consult: paroxysmal nocturnal hemoglobinuria and its complications. Blood 2013;122(16):2795–8.
74. Brodsky RA, Luznik L, Bolaños-Meade J, et al. Reduced intensity HLA-haploidentical BMT with post transplantation cyclophosphamide in nonmalignant hematologic diseases. Bone Marrow Transplant 2008;42(8):523–7.
75. Suenaga K, Kanda Y, Niiya H, et al. Successful application of nonmyeloablative transplantation for paroxysmal nocturnal hemoglobinuria. Exp Hematol 2001; 29(5):639–42.
76. Risitano AM, Notaro R, Marando L, et al. Complement fraction 3 binding on erythrocytes as additional mechanism of disease in paroxysmal nocturnal hemoglobinuria patients treated by eculizumab. Blood 2009;113:4094–100.
77. Botto M, Walport MJ. Hereditary deficiency of C3 in animals and humans. Int Rev Immunol 1993;10(1):37–50.
78. Lindorfer MA, Pawluczkowycz AW, Peek EM, et al. A novel approach to preventing the hemolysis of paroxysmal nocturnal hemoglobinuria: both complement-mediated cytolysis and C3 deposition are blocked by a monoclonal antibody specific for the alternative pathway of complement. Blood 2010;115(11):2283–91.
79. Sahu A, Soulika AM, Morikis D, et al. Binding kinetics, structure-activity relationship, and biotransformation of the complement inhibitor compstatin. J Immunol 2000;165(5):2491–9.

80. Sahu A, Lambris JD. Complement inhibitors: a resurgent concept in anti-inflammatory therapeutics. Immunopharmacology 2000;49(1–2):133–48.

81. Ricklin D, Lambris JD. Compstatin: a complement inhibitor on its way to clinical application. Adv Exp Med Biol 2008;632:273–92.

82. Risitano AM, Patrizia R, Caterina P, et al. Novel complement modulators for paroxysmal nocturnal hemoglobinuria: peptide and protein inhibitors of C3 convertase prevent both surface C3 deposition and subsequent hemolysis of affected erythrocytes in vitro. Blood (ASH Annual Meeting Abstracts) 2012;120:370.

83. Risitano AM, Ricklin D, Huang Y, et al. Peptide inhibitors of C3 activation as a novel strategy of complement inhibition for the treatment of paroxysmal nocturnal hemoglobinuria. Blood 2014;123(13):2094–101.

84. Cai S, Dole VS, Bergmeier W, et al. A direct role for C1 inhibitor in regulation of leukocyte adhesion. J Immunol 2005;174(10):6462–6.

85. Beinrohr L, Harmat V, Dobó J, et al. C1 inhibitor serpin domain structure reveals the likely mechanism of heparin potentiation and conformational disease. J Biol Chem 2007;282(29):21100–9.

86. DeZern AE, Uknis M, Yuan X, et al. Complement Blockade with a C1 Esterase Inhibitor in Paroxysmal Nocturnal Hemoglobinuria. Exp Hematol 2014;42:857–61.e1.

87. Hillmen P, Elebute M, Kelly R, et al. Long-term effect of the complement inhibitor eculizumab on kidney function in patients with paroxysmal nocturnal hemoglobinuria. Am J Hematol 2010;85(8):553–9.

88. Ferreira VP, Pangburn MK. Factor H mediated cell surface protection from complement is critical for the survival of PNH erythrocytes. Blood 2007;110(6):2190–2.

89. Whaley K, Ruddy S. Modulation of the alternative complement pathways by beta 1 H globulin. J Exp Med 1976;144(5):1147–63.

90. Risitano AM, Notaro R, Pascariello C, et al. The complement receptor 2/factor H fusion protein TT30 protects paroxysmal nocturnal hemoglobinuria erythrocytes from complement-mediated hemolysis and C3 fragment. Blood 2012;119(26):6307–16.

91. Schmidt CQ, Bai H, Lin Z, et al. Rational engineering of a minimized immune inhibitor with unique triple-targeting properties. J Immunol 2013;190(11):5712–21.

Congenital CD59 Deficiency

Britta Höchsmann, MD[a,b],*, Hubert Schrezenmeier, MD[a,b]

KEYWORDS

- CD59 deficiency • Glycosylphosphatidylinositol anchor
- Paroxysmal nocturnal hemoglobinuria • Terminal complement system
- Membrane attack complex inhibitory factor • Homologous restriction factor
- Membrane inhibitor of reactive lysis

KEY POINTS

- Congenital isolated deficiency of CD59, a key regulator of the complement system, is a rare disorder.
- Congenital isolated deficiency of CD59 is associated with Coombs-negative hemolysis and peripheral polyneuropathy.
- Flow cytometric analysis of expression of CD59 and other glycosylphosphatidylinositol-anchored proteins is an important step in diagnostic workup if CD59 deficiency is suspected.
- Targeted complement inhibition might become a new treatment option for congenital isolated deficiency of CD59.

INTRODUCTION

Homologous restriction factor (HRF 20), membrane inhibitor of reactive lysis (MIRL), membrane attack complex inhibitory factor (MACIF), protectin, and CD59 are a few of the many names for the same protein that was discovered when lysis of erythrocytes by complement in a homologous test system was studied. CD59 is a complement regulatory protein with a length of 128 amino acids that is attached to the cell surface by a glycosylphosphatidylinositol (GPI) anchor. GPI-anchored proteins exert multiple functions; some are important regulators of the complement system. The model disorder for a complement-mediated hemolytic anemia, paroxysmal nocturnal

Dr B. Höchsmann and Dr H. Schrezenmeier have received research funding and honraria by the pharmaceutic industry for PNH activities.

[a] Institute of Transfusion Medicine, University of Ulm, Ulm, Germany; [b] Institute of Clinical Transfusion Medicine and Immunogenetics Ulm, German Red Cross Blood Transfusion Service, Baden-Württemberg-Hessen, University Hospital of Ulm, Helmholtzstraße 10, Ulm 89081, Germany

* Corresponding author. Institute of Transfusion Medicine, University of Ulm, Helmholtzstraße 10, 89081 Ulm, Germany.

E-mail address: b.hoechsmann@blutspende.de

hemoglobinuria (PNH), is caused by a deficiency of all GPI-anchored proteins (including CD59) on the affected cells. PNH is caused by acquired *PIGA* gene mutations in hematopoietic stem cells, which cause a defect of the biosynthesis of the GPI-anchor.[1,2] Recently, a case of PNH caused by a germline splice site mutation of *PIGT* and an acquired deletion of *PIGT* in hematopoietic cells was reported.[3,4] This finding shows that genes that are essential for GPI biosynthesis and anchoring other than *PIGA* might also cause PNH. The frequency of these non-*PIGA* PNH cases still needs to be determined.[3,4]

In contrast to the acquired PNH, in which only hematopoietic cells harbor the *PIGA* mutation, in the rare inherited GPI-deficiency syndromes, all cells are affected. So far, underlying germline mutations were identified in *PIGL*,[5] *PIGM*,[6] *PIGN*,[7] *PIGO*,[8] *PIGT*,[9] *PIGV*,[10] and even CD59.[11,12] Additionally a germline *PIGA* gene mutation was recently reported in several families.[13-16] In PNH and the inherited defects of GPI anchor synthesis, the expression of the whole class of GPI-anchored proteins, including CD59, on the cell surface is affected. In contrast, isolated deficiency of CD59 is caused by inherited mutations in the CD59 gene. The biosynthesis of the GPI anchor itself and the expression of the other GPI-anchored proteins are normal. This disorder is rare. Only 7 cases have been published so far. Nevertheless, it gives important insight to the pathophysiologic role of CD59. Here, we review the genetic basis, differential diagnosis, clinical findings, and new treatment options for isolated inherited CD59 deficiency.

FUNCTION OF CD59

CD59 is a glycoprotein of approximately 20 kDa. It is attached by a GPI anchor to the membrane of many different cell types, including hematopoietic cells, endothelial cells, neurons, Schwann cells, oligodendrocytes, and astrocytes.[17] CD59 occurs at low concentration in soluble form in plasma, urine, and other body secretions. CD59 is a key regulator of the complement system and prevents complement attack by the inhibition of the membrane attack complex (MAC). The MAC triggers cell activation, endothelial damage, and cytotoxicity and leads to neurodegeneration and to cell lysis by the formation of a transmembrane pore (**Fig. 1**).

This pore is built by a complex of complement components C5b, C6, C7, and C8 (C5b-8) completed by a poly C9 complex consisting of 12 to 16 polymerized C9 molecules (poly C9).[18,19] This poly C9 can form tubular structures and can be inserted in phospholipid bilayers. However, poly C9 by itself is not cytolytic without a fully assembled MAC that is capable of forming channels through lipid bilayers.[18]

CD59 is the inhibitor of this reaction by binding to C9 or C5b-8, which reduces the development of poly C9. Therefore, a loss of CD59 increases the amount of poly C9 and consequently of the C5b-9 complexes, which leads to more functional transmembrane pores, resulting in an increase of osmotic cell lysis (**Fig. 2**).

Results of several studies point to the role of MAC and CD59 in causing demyelination and neuronal death in neurodegeneration. A CD59 deficit seems to be associated with the neuritic losses characteristic of Alzheimer's disease[20] and enhances disease severity, demyelination, and axonal injury in allergic encephalomyelitis.[21] Experimental data show that MAC formation provokes seizures and neurodegeneration.[22] In a mouse model of neuropathy, MAC deposits on damaged nerve terminal axons and surrounding perisynaptic Schwann cells were found.[23] Furthermore, damage is exacerbated in tissues from mice lacking CD59, in which MAC formation is increased.[24] CD59a knockout models in mice suggest that CD59a protects against ischemic brain damage[25] and mediates protection from secondary neuronal death after traumatic brain injury.[26]

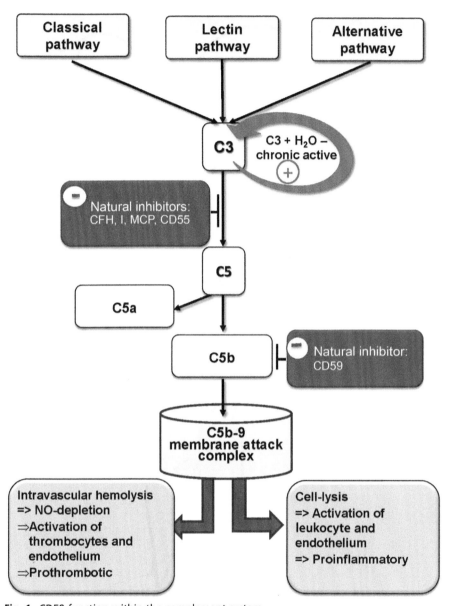

Fig. 1. CD59 function within the complement system.

CD59a and CD59b double-knockout in mice results in complement-mediated hemolysis and hemoglobinuria,[27] which can be rescued by deficiency of C3.[28,29]

GENETIC BASIS OF CD59 DEFICIENCY

So far, 3 different CD59 null alleles have been described. One patient from Japan carried the 2 single-base deletions c.123delC and c.361delG leading to a frameshift mutation with a stop codon at amino acid 38 (p.Val42Serfs*38; p.Ala121Glnfs).[11,12] Five CD59-deficient children originating from 4 unrelated North-African Jewish

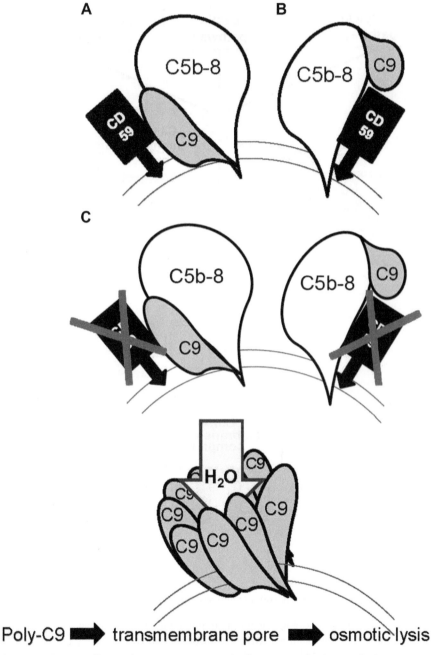

Fig. 2. Mechanism of CD59 function preventing the formation of poly C9, which is necessary to build a complete C5b-9 complex (MAC). (*A*) CD59 binds directly to C9. (*B*) CD59 binds to the C5b-8 complex limiting the number of C9 molecules interacting with C5b-8. (*C*) absent CD59 increases formation of complete C5b-9 complexes (MACs). ▒, Target protein expression in the sample; ☐, isotype control.

families all harbored the nucleotide substitution c.266G> A (p.Cys89Tyr), which likely is a founder mutation in Jews of North African ancestry.[30] The authors recently reported an isolated complete CD59 defect caused by the homozygous deletion c.146delA leading to a terminating codon at amino acid 31(p.Asp49Valfs*31) in a patient originating from Turkey.[31] The Japanese and the Turkish patient probably generate no functional protein. The altered protein of the North African patients was present in cells but absent on membranes. It is speculated that the changed tertiary structure may prevent the presentation of the altered protein on the membrane.[30]

CLINICAL SYMPTOMS OF CD59 DEFICIENCY

Except the single Japanese patient who was affected by the first hemolytic episode not before the age of 13, all 6 patients from North African and Turkish origin showed an early onset of the disease with 3 to 7 months. All published CD59-deficient individuals were severely ill and presented with recurrent hemolytic crises (**Table 1**).[11,12,30,31] Furthermore, a part of the complications observed in congenital CD59 deficiencies, like acute renal failure and thromboembolic events, are probably mediated by intravascular hemolysis. Reduction of availability of nitric oxide (NO) is a well-known mechanism in intravascular hemolysis, especially in PNH.[32] This reduction is caused by a disturbed synthesis and an increased consumption of NO.[32] Reduced bioavailability of NO results in platelet activation, endothelial dysfunction, and contraction of the vessels.[33] The Japanese patient suffered from 2 cerebral infarctions. In the Turkish child, diffusion disturbances suggestive of an ischemic stroke could be detected by cerebral MRI during the second hemolytic crisis. Thus, similar to acquired PNH, in inherited CD59 deficiency, the risk of thromboembolic complications might be increased. Symptoms involving the peripheral nervous system were reported in all published cases except the Japanese patient published by Yamashina and colleagues (see **Table 1**).[11,12,30,31] In most cases, the neurologic symptoms are more prominent than the hemolysis, which only becomes clinically relevant during episodes of complement activation, especially during infections. The mechanism behind this observation seems to be the limited neuronal capacity of controlling complement activation because of low neuronal CD59 expression.

The common feature in these 6 individuals with a congenital CD59 deficiency and neurologic symptoms is a generalized progressive muscular hypotonia with flaccid paralysis, presenting like a chronic inflammatory demyelinating polyradiculoneuropathy.[30,31] One patient showed, in addition, symptoms of the central nerve system (bulbar symptoms, ie, inability to swallow, abducens, and facial nerve palsy) and focal seizures.[31]

The reason for differences in clinical presentation is currently unknown, and more cases may be necessary to draw definite conclusions. A comparison of the clinical characteristics of the cases is listed in **Table 1**.

LABORATORY DIAGNOSIS OF CD59 DEFICIENCY

Acquired CD59 deficiency caused by a GPI-anchor defect on hematopoietic cells is a hallmark of PNH. Varying percentages of hematopoietic cells are affected, and PNH is characterized by a mosaic of cells with normal and absent or reduced expression of GPI-anchored proteins.

In contrast to PNH, which affect the synthesis of the GPI anchor and, therefore, the expression of all GPI-anchored proteins on the cell surfaces, only CD59 expression is missing in congenital CD59 deficiency, and the defect is not confined to hematopoietic cells.

Table 1
Published cases with congenital CD59 deficiency and their characteristics

Ethnic Origin	Congenital CD59 Deficiency		
	Japanese	Turkish	North African Jewish
Number of patients	1, parents consanguineous	1, parents consanguineous	5; from 4 parents consanguineous
Location of mutation	Frameshift mutation leading to terminating codon at amino acid 38 (p.Val42Serfs*38; p.Ala121Glnfs)	Frameshift mutation leading to terminating codon at amino acid 31 (c.146delA, pAsp49Valfs*31)	Homozygous missense mutation leading to amino acid substitution from Cys to Tyr in position 89 (p.Cys89Tyr)
Onset of disease	13 y	7 mo	3–7 mo
Hemolysis	Yes	Yes	Yes
Thrombo-embolic events	Yes, cerebral infarction	MRI suggestive of ischemic stroke during the second hemolytic crisis	No
Neurologic disease	Nothing reported (beside the cerebral infarctions)	Progressive neurologic impairment: focal seizures, bulbar symptoms, abducens and facial nerve palsy; generalized muscular hypotonia (legs flaccid and muscle reflexes absent), ventilation required	Relapsing polyneuropathy, presenting as chronic inflammatory demyelinating polyradiculoneuropathy with symmetric muscle weakness, accompanied by hypotonia and absent tendon reflexes involving the legs > arms
Treatment	Nothing reported	Immunoglobulins intravenously; plasmapheresis, transfusions without response; Eculizumab, with treatment response of hemolysis and neurologic symptoms	Immunoglobulins intravenously, plasmapheresis, corticosteroid, rituximab, and cyclosporine did not prevent recurrences but seemed to have effect on relapses length and severity
Reference	Yamashina et al,[11] 1990 Motoyama et al,[12] 1992	Höchsmann et al,[31] 2014	Nevo et al,[30] 2013

Flow cytometric screening for PNH is mandatory in workup of hemolytic anemia with a negative Coombs test result (direct antiglobulin test). The screening panel should consist of a minimum of 2 different GPI-anchored markers (including CD59) on a minimum of 2 different cell lines.[33–36] Screening with a single marker (eg, based on CD55 or CD16 alone) would have missed the diagnosis in these cases of isolated CD59 deficiency (**Fig. 3**). On the other hand, screening with CD59 as a single marker could have suggested the wrong diagnosis of acquired PNH.

The authors recommend the following diagnostic steps if isolated CD59 deficiency is suspected:

- First, the CD59 expression has to be tested at least on erythrocytes and granulocytes. In addition, monocytes and lymphocytes can be studied.
- Other GPI-anchored markers (eg, CD55 or CD58 on red cells or CD16, CD24, CD66b, or CD157 on granulocytes) need to be analyzed to distinguish isolated CD59 deficiency from PNH, which is characterized by concordant deficiency of all GPI-anchored markers and the GPI anchor itself. The latter can be tested by the fluorescein-labeled proaerolysin, a bacterial toxin that specifically binds to the GPI anchor test.
- If an isolated CD59 deficiency is verified in all examined cell lines, the suspected diagnosis should be confirmed by sequencing of the CD59 gene.
- This is also true for cases of a cell population with reduced, but not completely absent, CD59 expression, as such a pattern has been reported in heterozygous carriers.

Genetic analysis of suspected heterozygous carriers might be important even in absence of clinical symptoms for genetic counseling.

The intravascular hemolysis might result in clinical complications similar to those of PNH. Therefore, the authors recommend that diagnostic workup be done as in PNH with regard to thromboembolic events, renal function disturbance, deficiency of iron, deficiency of folic acid, deficiency of vitamin B12, pulmonary hypertension, arterial hypertension, abdominal pain, and hemoglobinuria. Laboratory work should include, at a minimum, complete blood count, reticulocytes, lactate dehydrogenase, haptoglobin, creatinine, direct antiglobulin test, and screen for CD59 antibodies (see later discussion). Furthermore signs and symptoms of the peripheral and central nervous systems have to be evaluated by anamnesis and physical examination. Additionally, measurement of motor nerve conduction velocity is helpful to assess the impairment of the peripheral nervous system at the initial diagnosis and during the course of the disease.

The reported cases should increase awareness for inherited CD59 deficiency. Although neurologic symptoms or hemolysis seem to be an indication of inherited CD59 deficiency, the presentation can vary (see **Table 1**). Also inherited deficiencies of GPI anchor synthesis caused by *PIGM, PIGA, PIGL, PIGO, PIGN*, or *PIGV* gene mutations need to be considered as differential diagnosis. Early diagnosis of congenital CD59 deficiency becomes even more important because now there might be an option for targeted therapy.[31]

CD59 AS A BLOOD GROUP

Recently, CD59 was identified as a new blood group antigen because of the detection of an anti-CD59 alloantibody in the Turkish patient with a congenital homozygous CD59 mutation.[31,37]

The International Society of Blood Transfusion established criteria for constituting a new blood group system: the blood group antigen is defined by a human

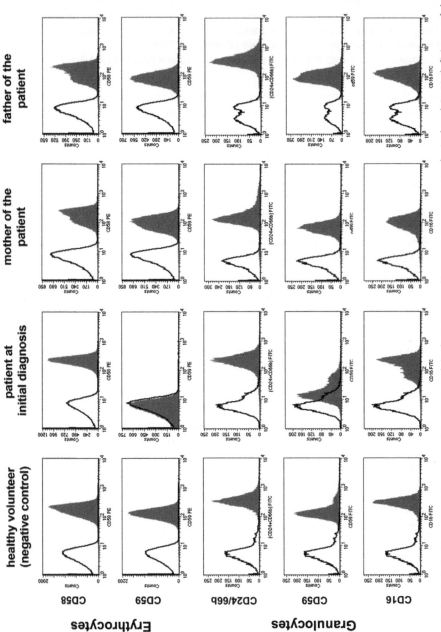

Fig. 3. Flow cytometric detection of GPI-AP expression patterns of the heterozygous parents. In contrast to the isolated CD59 deficiency of the patient, CD59 is still expressed on erythrocytes and granulocytes of the heterozygous parents. (*From Supplement to* Höchsmann B, Dohna-Schwake C, Kyrieleis H, et al. Targeted therapy with Eculizumab for inherited CD59 deficiency. N Engl J Med 2014;370(Suppl 1):56; with permission.)

alloantibody[37] and is inherited.[31] The encoding gene is sequenced, is different from other blood group genes, and its chromosomal location is known.[38–40] All these criteria are fulfilled, and the International Society of Blood Transfusion working party for red cell immunogenetics and blood group nomenclature approved CD59 as a new blood group system.[41] The new system currently comprises 1 antigen and 3 null alleles.[37,41]

If a red cell alloantibody is detected in the antibody screen in a patient with known or suspected CD59 deficiency, it should be considered that it is an anti-CD59 alloantibody, in particular if the patient had received previous blood transfusions. In the CD59-deficient patient, the antibody could be easily identified in the plasma by an inhibition test using soluble recombinant CD59.[37]

The time point of alloimmunization in that child is not clearly defined, but the CD59 antibody had decreased to almost undetectable levels 2 years after the last transfusion. CD59 represents an antigen that is highly expressed on the red cells. Despite this fact, no major adverse clinical signs of a transfusion reaction were evident in the transfusion history of this patient.[37]

Thus, the question of clinical relevance of an anti-CD59 alloantibody is currently not clear. However, we recommend a restrictive transfusion regime. The CD59 antibody titer should be controlled in CD59-deficient patients before and after transfusions, if a transfusion is not avoidable.

In case of the need for transfusions, one might use the blood of heterozygous carriers who showed a lower CD59 expression on the red blood cells.[37] On the other hand, the higher immunization risk by using blood products of family members has to be considered. If blood products of family members are chosen, the products have to be irradiated.

CD59 DEFICIENCY AND TREATMENT

Until now, therapeutic approaches for inherited GPI deficiencies were limited. Only the histone deacetylase inhibitor, sodium butyrate, was shown as an effective therapy in inherited GPI deficiency caused by a mutation in the *PIGM* core promoter. So far, no specific treatment for inherited CD59 deficiency has been reported.[6] Immunosuppressive approaches like corticosteroid, rituximab, and cyclosporine did not protect against recurrences.[30,31]

This lack of established specific treatment options and the progressive clinical worsening of the patient led to off-label use of the C5 antibody, eculizumab, an inhibitor of the terminal complement system in the Turkish case.[31] Basis for this treatment approach is the known function of CD59 as a MAC inhibitor and the presumably insufficient prevention of complement attack in congenital CD59 deficiency. Based on the experience in PNH,[42–44] we expected that eculizumab might reduce the complement-mediated hemolysis and the related complications, like thromboembolic events and renal insufficiency, and also might stop further MAC-induced cell damage, even on neuronal cells.

These considerations were supported by data in animals and humans indicating a positive influence of complement inhibition on various neurologic disorders.[45–51] Halstead and colleagues and others[45–48] reported that inhibition of complement activation rescued the integrity of axonal and perisynaptic Schwann cells in antiganglioside antibody-mediated neuropathy. Additionally, an influence of the MAC and the complement activation in regeneration processes after nerve trauma and stroke has been reported.[47,51] Furthermore, recent publications show data confirming the C5 antibody, eculizumab, as a therapy option for patients suffering from neuromyelitis optica when complement activation and MAC formation destroys astrocytes and generalized myasthenia gravis.[49,50]

Our hypothesis was clinically confirmed by a reduction of hemolysis after the first eculizumab infusions—similar to PNH treatment. Furthermore, progression of neurologic symptoms (focal seizures, bulbar symptoms, generalized muscular hypotonia, and need for ventilation) stopped. More than expected, not only stabilization but also improvement of neurologic symptoms and objective parameters such as motoneuron conductive velocity, was observed. The first signs of this neurologic benefit were seen about 6 months after starting eculizumab, and after 30 months a remarkable continuous improvement was reported. The patient no longer had bulbar symptoms, had no need for ventilation or a stomach tube, can eat and swallow, and is able to stand up for a short time.[31]

The inhibition of the terminal complement system and MAC formation stopped further nerval damage and seemed to support neuronal regeneration in this case. Therefore, one might speculate whether an earlier onset of eculizumab treatment could have avoided progressive neurologic damage and the irreversible visual impairment of the patient. Investigation of eculizumab use in further patients with congenital CD59 deficiency is necessary to finally assess its benefit in this disorder.

In addition to this new specific treatment option, supportive treatment is also necessary. This treatment includes early and definitive treatment of infections to prevent strong complement activation and consecutive hemolytic crises, hydration during hemolytic crises to avoid renal damage, and prophylactic anticoagulation during hemolytic crises. Substitution of iron, folic acid, and B vitamins should be performed if required. Physiotherapy is an important part of the treatment in patients with symptoms of the peripheral nerve system to avoid muscle reduction.

SUMMARY

The recent findings of germline mutations in *PIGL*,[5] *PIGN*,[7] *PIGO*,[8] *PIGT*,[9] *PIGV*,[10] *CD59*[11,12] and even *PIGA*,[13] suggest a wide phenotypic spectrum of disorders that affect either the biosynthesis of the GPI anchor itself or the specific GPI-anchored protein CD59 with or without hemolysis. Common clinical presentations are neurologic symptoms in inherited isolated CD59 deficiency, in particular, a progressive muscular hypotonia with flaccid paralysis mimicking CIPD. Congenital deficiency of CD59 seems to be an ultra rare disorder. However, it must be considered in children with unclear neurologic symptoms and hemolysis (which might occur only transiently). Detection of isolated CD59 deficiency and distinction from other GPI anchor disorders (PNH, congenital GPI-pathway disorders) can easily be performed by flow cytometry.

The severe clinical symptoms of inherited CD59 deficiency confirm the importance of CD59 as essential complement regulatory protein for protection of cells against complement attack, in particular, protection of human neuronal tissue. Targeted complement inhibition might become a treatment option as suggested by a case report.[31] The easy diagnostic approach by flow cytometry and the advent of a new treatment option should increase the awareness of this rare differential diagnosis and lead to further studies on their pathophysiology.

REFERENCES

1. Miyata T, Yamada N, Iida Y, et al. Abnormalities of PIG-A transcripts in granulocytes from patients with paroxysmal nocturnal hemoglobinuria. N Engl J Med 1994;330(4):249–55.
2. Hillmen P, Lewis SM, Bessler M, et al. Natural history of paroxysmal nocturnal hemoglobinuria. N Engl J Med 1995;333(19):1253–8.

3. Krawitz PM, Höchsmann B, Murakami Y, et al. A case of paroxysmal nocturnal hemoglobinuria caused by a germline mutation and a somatic mutation in PIGT. Blood 2013;122(7):1312–5.
4. Luzzatto L. PNH from mutations of another PIG gene. Blood 2013;122(7): 1099–100.
5. Ng BG, Hackmann K, Jones MA, et al. Mutations in the glycosylphosphatidylinositol gene PIGL cause CHIME syndrome. Am J Hum Genet 2012;90(4):685–8.
6. Almeida AM, Murakami Y, Baker A, et al. Targeted therapy for inherited GPI deficiency. N Engl J Med 2007;356(16):1641–7.
7. Maydan G, Noyman I, Har-Zahav A, et al. Multiple congenital anomalies-hypotonia-seizures syndrome is caused by a mutation in PIGN. J Med Genet 2011;48(6):383–9.
8. Krawitz PM, Murakami Y, Hecht J, et al. Mutations in PIGO, a member of the GPI-anchor-synthesis pathway, cause hyperphosphatasia with mental retardation. Am J Hum Genet 2012;91(1):146–51.
9. Kvarnung M, Nilsson D, Lindstrand A, et al. A novel intellectual disability syndrome caused by GPI anchor deficiency due to homozygous mutations in PIGT. J Med Genet 2013;50(8):521–8.
10. Krawitz PM, Schweiger MR, Rodelsperger C, et al. Identity-by-descent filtering of exome sequence data identifies PIGV mutations in hyperphosphatasia mental retardation syndrome. Nat Genet 2010;42(10):827–9.
11. Yamashina M, Ueda E, Kinoshita T, et al. Inherited complete deficiency of 20-kilodalton homologous restriction factor (CD59) as a cause of paroxysmal nocturnal hemoglobinuria. N Engl J Med 1990;323(17):1184–9.
12. Motoyama N, Okada N, Yamashina M, et al. Paroxysmal nocturnal hemoglobinuria due to hereditary nucleotide deletion in the HRF20 (CD59) gene. Eur J Immunol 1992;22(10):2669–73.
13. Johnston JJ, Gropman AL, Sapp JC, et al. The phenotype of a germline mutation in PIGA: the gene somatically mutated in paroxysmal nocturnal hemoglobinuria. Am J Hum Genet 2012;90(2):295–300.
14. van der Crabben SN, Harakalova M, Brilstra EH, et al. Expanding the spectrum of phenotypes associated with germline PIGA mutations: a child with developmental delay, accelerated linear growth, facial dysmorphisms, elevated alkaline phosphatase, and progressive CNS abnormalities. Am J Med Genet A 2014; 164A(1):29–35.
15. Belet S, Fieremans N, Yuan X, et al. Early frameshift mutation in PIGA identified in a large XLID family without neonatal lethality. Hum Mutat 2014;35(3): 350–5.
16. Swoboda KJ, Margraf RL, Carey JC, et al. A novel germline PIGA mutation in Ferro-Cerebro-Cutaneous syndrome: a neurodegenerative X-linked epileptic encephalopathy with systemic iron-overload. Am J Med Genet 2014;164A(1):17–28.
17. Vedeler C, Ulvestad E, Bjorge L, et al. The expression of CD59 in normal human nervous tissue. Immunology 1994;82(4):542–7.
18. Podack ER, Tschoop J, Muller-Eberhard HJ. Molecular organization of C9 within the membrane attack complex of complement. Induction of circular C9 polymerization by the C5b-8 assembly. J Exp Med 1982;156(1):268–82.
19. Kolb WP, Haxby JA, Arroyave CM, et al. Molecular analysis of the membrane attack mechanism of complement. J Exp Med 1972;135(3):549–66.
20. Yang LB, Li R, Meri S, et al. Deficiency of complement defense protein CD59 may contribute to neurodegeneration in Alzheimer's disease. J Neurosci 2000;20(20): 7505–9.

21. Mead RJ, Neal JW, Griffiths MR, et al. Deficiency of the complement regulator CD59a enhances disease severity, demyelination and axonal injury in murine acute experimental allergic encephalomyelitis. Lab Invest 2004;84(1):21–8.
22. Xiong ZQ, Qian W, Suzuki K, et al. Formation of complement membrane attack complex in mammalian cerebral cortex evokes seizures and neurodegeneration. J Neurosci 2003;23(3):955–60.
23. Singhrao SK, Neal JW, Rushmere NK, et al. Spontaneous classical pathway activation and deficiency of membrane regulators render human neurons susceptible to complement lysis. Am J Pathol 2000;157(3):905–18.
24. Halstead SK, O'Hanlon GM, Humphreys PD, et al. Anti-disialoside antibodies kill perisynaptic schwann cells and damage motor nerve terminals via membrane attack complex in a murine model of neuropathy. Brain 2004;127(9):2109–23.
25. Harhausen D, Khojasteh U, Stahel PF, et al. Membrane attack complex inhibitor CD59a protects against focal cerebral ischemia in mice. J Neuroinflammation 2010;7:15.
26. Stahel PF, Flierl MA, Morgan BP, et al. Absence of the complement regulatory molecule CD59a leads to exacerbated neuropathology after traumatic brain injury in mice. J Neuroinflammation 2009;6:2.
27. Holt DS, Botto M, Bygrave AE, et al. Targeted deletion of the CD59 gene causes spontaneous intravascular hemolysis and hemoglobinuria. Blood 2001;98(2):442–9.
28. Qin X, Dobarro M, Bedford SJ, et al. Further characterization of reproductive abnormalities in mCd59b knockout mice: a potential new function of mCd59 in male reproduction. J Immunol 2005;175(20):6294–302.
29. Baalasubramanian S, Harris CL, Donev RM, et al. CD59a is the primary regulator of membrane attack complex assembly in the mouse. J Immunol 2004;173(6):3684–92.
30. Nevo Y, Ben-Zeev B, Tabib A, et al. CD59 deficiency is associated with chronic hemolysis and childhood relapsing immune mediated polyneuropathy. Blood 2013;121(1):129–35.
31. Höchsmann B, Dohna-Schwake C, Kyrieleis H, et al. Targeted therapy with Eculizumab for inherited CD59 deficiency. N Engl J Med 2014;370(1):90–2.
32. Hill A, Rother RP, Wang X, et al. Effect of eculizumab on haemolysis-associated nitric oxide depletion, dyspnoea, and measures of pulmonary hypertension in patients with paroxysmal nocturnal haemoglobinuria. Br J Haematol 2010;149(3):414–25.
33. Hill A, Kelly RJ, Hillmen P. Thrombosis in paroxysmal nocturnal hemoglobinuria. Blood 2013;121(25):4985–96 [quiz: 5105].
34. Borowitz MJ, Craig FE, Digiuseppe JA, et al. Guidelines for the diagnosis and monitoring of paroxysmal nocturnal hemoglobinuria and related disorders by flow cytometry. Cytometry B Clin Cytom 2010;78(4):211–30.
35. Schrezenmeier H, Bettelheim P, Panse J, et al. Recommendations for the diagnosis of paroxysmal nocturnal hemoglobinuria: a German-Austrian consensus. J Lab Med 2012;35(6):1439–77.
36. Höchsmann B, Rojewski M, Schrezenmeier H. Paroxysmal nocturnal hemoglobinuria (PNH): higher sensitivity and validity in diagnosis and serial monitoring by flow cytometric analysis of reticulocytes. Ann Hematol 2011;90(8):887–99.
37. Anliker M, von Zabern I, Höchsmann B, et al. A new blood group antigen is defined by anti-CD59, detected in a CD59-deficient patient. Transfusion 2014;54(7):1817–22.

38. Meri S, Lehto T, Sutton CW, et al. Structural composition and functional character-ization of soluble CD59: heterogeneity of the oligosaccharide and glycophos-phoinositol (GPI) anchor revealed by laser-desorption mass spectrometric analysis. Biochem J 1996;316(Pt 3):923–35.

39. Huang Y, Fedarovich A, Tomlinson S, et al. Crystal structure of CD59: implications for molecular recognition of the complement proteins C8 and C9 in the membrane-attack complex. Acta Crystallogr D Biol Crystallogr 2007;63(Pt 6): 714–21.

40. Forsberg UH, Bazil V, Stefanová I, et al. Gene for human CD59 (likely Ly-6 homo-logoue) is located on the short arm of chromosome 11. Immunogenetics 1989; 30(3):188–93.

41. Storry JR. International society of blood transfusion working party on red cell immunogenetics and blood group terminology: cancun report (2012). Vox Sang 2014;107(1):90–6.

42. Hillmen P, Young NS, Schubert J, et al. The complement inhibitor eculizumab in paroxysmal nocturnal hemoglobinuria. N Engl J Med 2006;355(12):1233–43.

43. Kelly RJ, Hill A, Arnold LM, et al. Long-term treatment with eculizumab in parox-ysmal nocturnal hemoglobinuria: sustained efficacy and improved survival. Blood 2011;117(25):6786–92.

44. Höchsmann B, Leichtle R, von Zabern I, et al. Paroxysmal nocturnal haemoglobi-nuria treatment with eculizumab is associated with a positive direct antiglobulin test. Vox Sang 2012;102(2):159–66.

45. Halstead SK, Humphreys PD, Goodfellow JA, et al. Complement inhibition abro-gates nerve terminal injury in miller fisher syndrome. Ann Neurol 2005;58(2): 203–10.

46. Kolev MV, Tediose T, Sivanskar B, et al. Upregulating CD59: a new strategy for protection of neurons from complement-mediated degeneration. Pharmacogenomics 2010;10(1):12–9.

47. Arumugam TV, Woodruff TM, Lathia JD, et al. Neuroprotection in stroke by com-plement inhibition and immunoglobulin therapy. Neuroscience 2009;158(3): 1074–89.

48. Halstead SK, Zitman FM, Humphreys PD, et al. Eculizumab prevents anti-ganglioside antibody-mediated neuropathy in a murine model. Brain 2008; 131(Pt 5):1197–208.

49. Howard J, Barohn R, Freimer M, et al. Randomized, double-blind, placebo-controlled, crossover, multicenter, phase II study of eculizumab in patients with refractory generalized myasthenia gravis (gMG). Neurology 2012;78 [Meeting abstract: S35.004].

50. Pittock SJ, Lennon VA, McKeon A, et al. Eculizumab in AQP4-IgG-positive relaps-ing neuromyelitis optica spectrum disorders: an open-label pilot study. Lancet Neurol 2013;12(6):554–62.

51. Ramaglia V, Wolterman R, de Kok M, et al. Soluble complement receptor 1 protects the peripheral nerve from early axon loss after injury. Am J Pathol 2008;172(4):1043–52.

Ultralarge Von Willebrand Factor–Induced Platelet Clumping and Activation of the Alternative Complement Pathway in Thrombotic Thrombocytopenic Purpura and the Hemolytic-Uremic Syndromes

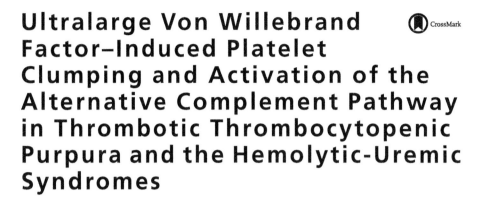

Nancy Turner, BA[a], Sarah Sartain, MD[a,b], Joel Moake, MD[a,*]

KEYWORDS

• VWF • Alternative complement pathway • Factor H • Thrombotic microangiopathies

KEY POINTS

- The molecular linkage between ultralarge (UL) von Willebrand factor (VWF) multimers and the alternative complement pathway (AP) has recently been described.
- Endothelial cell (EC)-secreted and anchored ULVWF multimers (in long stringlike structures) function as both hyperadhesive sites that initiate platelet adhesion and aggregation and activating surfaces for the AP.
- In vitro, the active form of C3, C3b binds to the EC-anchored ULVWF multimeric strings and initiates the assembly on the strings of C3 convertase (C3bBb) and C5 convertase (C3bBbC3b).
- In vivo, activation of the AP via this mechanism proceeds all the way to generation of terminal complement complexes (C5b-9).
- The linkage of EC-secreted and anchored ULVWF multimeric strings, excessive platelet adhesion/aggregation, and activation of the AP explains many of the clinical similarities among (1) severe ADAMTS-13 (a disintegrin and metalloprotease with thrombospondin domains, #13)-deficient thrombotic thrombocytopenic purpura (TTP); (2) TTP-like syndromes associated with only modest deficiencies of ADAMTS-13; (3) enterohemorrhagic *Escherichia coli*–associated hemolytic-uremic syndrome; and (4) the provocation of episodes of atypical HUS, which are associated with overactivation of the AP.

The authors have nothing to disclose.
This work was supported by grants from the Mary R. Gibson Foundation and the Mabel and Everett Hinkson Memorial Fund.
[a] Department of Bioengineering, Rice University, 6500 Main Street, Houston, TX 77030, USA;
[b] Section of Hematology-Oncology, Department of Pediatrics, Texas Children's Cancer and Hematology Centers, Baylor College of Medicine, 6701 Fannin St., Houston, TX 77004, USA
* Corresponding author.
E-mail address: jmoake@rice.edu

Hematol Oncol Clin N Am 29 (2015) 509–524
http://dx.doi.org/10.1016/j.hoc.2015.01.008
0889-8588/15/$ – see front matter © 2015 Elsevier Inc. All rights reserved.

THROMBOTIC MICROANGIOPATHIES (TMAS)

Common clinical characteristics of the thrombotic microangiopathies, thrombotic thrombocytopenic purpura (TTP), hemolytic-uremic syndromes associated with enterohemorrhagic *Escherichia coli* (EHEC-HUS), and atypical hemolytic-uremic syndrome (aHUS), include microvascular platelet adhesion/aggregation, thrombocytopenia, and erythrocyte fragmentation.[1] Excessive platelet adhesion/aggregation *and* activation of the alternative complement pathway (AP) on endothelial cells (EC)-secreted/anchored ultralarge (UL) von Willebrand factor (ULVWF) multimeric strings are involved in all of these syndromes.

Recent studies have demonstrated the precise molecular linkage between EC-secreted/anchored ULVWF multimers and activation of the alternative AP.[2] This linkage is likely to be of considerable clinical importance in the thrombotic microangiopathies, including TTP and the EHEC-HUS or with overactivation of the AP (aHUS).

OVERVIEW OF THE THROMBOTIC MICROANGIOPATHIES
A Disintegrin and Metalloprotease with Thrombospondin Domains, #13-Deficient Thrombotic Thrombocytopenic Purpura

During hemostasis and thrombosis, stimulated human vascular ECs secrete and anchor ULVWF multimers in hyperadhesive long stringlike structures that initiate platelet adhesion. Severe TTP is usually associated with less than 10% of plasma ADAMTS-13 (a disintegrin and metalloproteinase with a thrombospondin type-1 motif, member #13), the Ca^{2+}/Zn^{2+}-metalloprotease responsible for cleaving EC-secreted/anchored ULVWF multimeric strings. Severe ADAMTS-13 deficiency is caused by congenital homozygous or double-heterozygous *ADAMTS13* gene mutations, or by the acquired production of polyclonal autoantibodies directed against the spacer domain of the metalloprotease.[3–5] The result is little or no cleavage of EC-secreted/anchored ULVWF multimeric strings, excessive platelet adhesion/aggregation on the uncleaved hyperadhesive strings, and the formation of microvascular thrombi (**Figs. 1** and **2A, B**).

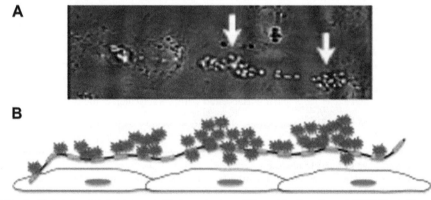

A

B

Fig. 1. Platelet adhesion/aggregation on human EC-secreted/anchored ULVWF multimeric strings in the presence of severe ADAMTS-13-deficient human plasma. (*A*) Phase contrast image of platelet attachment to EC-anchored ULVWF strings (*arrows*) after perfusion of normal washed platelets suspended in ADAMTS-13-deficient plasma (<10%) over histamine-stimulated ECs. (The few black particles shown are underlying cellular debris.) (*B*) Cartoon of thrombus formation on EC-secreted/anchored ULVWF strings under conditions of severe plasma ADAMTS-13-deficiency (<10%), as in congenital and anti-ADAMTS-13 autoantibody-mediated TTP.

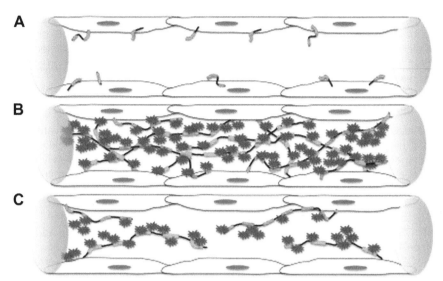

Fig. 2. Cartoon views of blood vessels showing varying amounts of uncleaved EC-anchored ULVWF string cleavage, and the associated extent of platelet adhesion/aggregation. (*A*) Normal levels of ADAMTS-13 activity; (*B*) severe deficiency (<10%) of functional ADAMTS-13; and (*C*) mild to modest ADAMTS-13-deficiency (>10%).

More modest deficiencies of ADAMTS-13 may also result in platelet adhesion/aggregation greater than normal in other thrombotic microangiopathies, as described in the sections to follow and depicted in **Fig. 2C.**

Enterohemorrhagic Escherichia coli–Associated Hemolytic-Uremic Syndrome

HUS is a leading cause of acute renal failure in children.[6,7] Most commonly, these HUS cases are associated with inadvertent ingestion of enterohemorrhagic *E coli* and are characterized by episodes of bloody diarrhea followed by the formation of occlusive glomerular platelet-fibrin thrombi.[1,7,8]

EHEC-HUS can also be acquired by ingestion of *Shigella dysenteriae* serotype 1, which is the prototype Shiga toxin microbe. More frequently, however, the causative organisms belong to one of several strains of enterohemorrhagic *E coli* (eg, O157:H7; or O104:H4 [in the 2011 European outbreak]).[9,10] These *E coli* strains produce Shiga-like toxin-1 (Stx-1) or Shiga-like toxin-2 (Stx-2).[1,8,11,12] These Shiga toxins are 70-kDa exotoxins, composed of 5 B subunits (7.7 kDa each) and an A subunit (composed of disulfide bonded chains of 28 and 4 kDa).[13,14] The B subunit mediates attachment and cellular entry through a membrane globotriaosylceramide receptor (Gb3 or CD77) present on ECs—and especially abundant on renal glomerular microvascular ECs. The A subunit is internalized and inhibits protein synthesis.[1,15,16]

Atypical Hemolytic-Uremic Syndrome

aHUS is a complication of excessive AP activation. Prominent causes of aHUS are a heterozygous mutation of the complement factor H (*CFH*) gene on chromosome 1; or homozygous deletion in genes for the CFH-related (CFHR)-1 and CFHR-3 proteins of the *CFH* gene cluster (chromosome 1) plus autoantibody-mediated inhibition of FH (deficiency of CFHR plasma proteins and autoantibody-positive HUS).[17–19] Other mutations associated with aHUS include heterozygous loss-of-function mutations in complement factor I (*CFI*, chromosome 4), in *CD46* (membrane cofactor protein; chromosome 1), or in *THBD* (thrombomodulin or CD141; chromosome 20). Heterozygous gain-of-function mutations in the *C3* gene (chromosome 19) or in the complement factor B gene (*CFB*; chromosome 6) have been associated with aHUS.[20,21] Excessive AP activity in aHUS results in damage or perturbation of renal ECs, resulting in episodes of acute renal failure.[22]

OVERVIEW OF THE ALTERNATIVE COMPLEMENT PATHWAY

The initiation of the AP requires an "activating surface" to cleave and activate C3 to C3b. The process of C3 cleavage generates C3a fragments ($\sim$9 kDa) with histamine-releasing and chemotactic activities. C3b attaches covalently via a cleavage-exposed thioester to carbohydrates or hydroxyl-containing amino acids (threonine, serine, and tyrosine) on activating surfaces.[23,24] Bound C3b then binds factor B (FB) to produce C3bB.[25,26] The FB in the C3bB complex is cleaved by factor D (FD) to form C3bBb, the AP C3 convertase that is stabilized by factor P (FP).[27–29] The Bb in C3bBb on an activating surface cleaves fluid-phase C3 to generate additional surface-bound C3b molecules and rapidly amplify the generation of C3b generation from C3. As the ratio of C3b to Bb increases, C3bBbC3b (the C5 convertase) is formed. C5 convertase binds C5 with high affinity and cleaves/activates C5 to C5b, releasing the peptide fragment, C5a ($\sim$10 kDa). C5a is similar to C3a in also possessing histamine-releasing and chemotactic activity.[30,31]

ULTRALARGE VON WILLEBRAND FACTOR MULTIMERS AND INITIATION OF THE ALTERNATIVE COMPLEMENT PATHWAY

It has been recently discovered[2] that AP initiation occurs on ULVWF multimeric strings that have been secreted by, and are anchored to, the surfaces of stimulated ECs. Human umbilical vein endothelial cells (HUVECs) and other ECs are miniature "factories" that express the mRNA for complement components and synthesize the associated proteins. In these in vitro experiments, there was no requirement for the addition of any additional purified components. Uncleaved ULVWF multimeric strings secreted by, and anchored to, stimulated ECs were found to be "activating surfaces" for C3b binding and AP assembly and activation (**Fig. 3**A, **Table 1**). C3 (as C3b), FB (as Bb), FD, FP, and C5 (as C5b), FH, and FI attached to EC-secreted and anchored ULVWF strings. In contrast, C4 (as C4b) did not attach to the ULVWF strings, indicating that the classical and lectin pathways were not activated (see **Fig 3**B, see **Table 1**). The attachment to EC-secreted/anchored ULVWF strings of C3b, Bb, and C5b occurred in quantitative and functional patterns consistent with the assembly of AP components into active complexes of C3 convertase (C3bBb) and C5 convertase (C3bBbC3b) (**Fig. 4**A).

The AP negative regulatory components, FH and FI, also bind to EC-secreted/anchored ULVWF strings. The extent of their binding is, however, about one-third less than the binding of C3b (see **Table 1**). FH and FI may, therefore, slow, but not prevent, EC-anchored ULVWF multimeric strings from gating C3 and C5 convertases.

These experiments established the molecular linkage between the AP and the earliest events in hemostasis-thrombosis (ie, the stimulation of vascular ECs to secrete and anchor ULVWF multimeric strings). In the in vitro studies summarized above, the AP was assembled and activated on ULVWF strings that were not rapidly cleaved because of inadequate ADAMTS-13 in the model system.[2] Inflammatory cytokines, bacterial toxins, phosphodiesterase inhibitors, calcium ionophore, and high concentrations of histamine are examples of agents that can cause EC stimulation and increase rates of EC secretion/anchorage of ULVWF strings in vitro.[8,32,33] Inflammatory cytokines

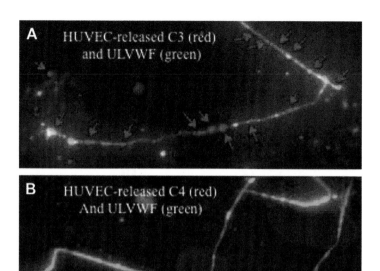

Fig. 3. Immunofluorescent microscopy images of EC-anchored ULVWF multimeric strings detecting (A) C3 (as C3b) and (B) C4 (as C4b). HUVECs stimulated for 2 minutes with 100 μM histamine were stained for 15 minutes with rabbit antihuman VWF antibody plus chicken antirabbit IgG-Alexa Fluor (AF)-488 (green) followed by the addition of fixative. The cells were then stained for C3 or C4 using monospecific goat antihuman antibodies plus secondary donkey antigoat IgG-AF-594 (red). Cell nuclei were detected with DAPI (4′,6-diamidino-2-phenylindole, blue). Combined images at ×600 are shown. The red arrows in (A) indicate some of the sites of C3b attachment onto a ULVWF string. There is no detectable attachment in this field of C4b to the ULVWF string, indicating a lack of activation of the classical and lectin complement pathways.

Table 1
Components of the alternative complement pathway attached to endothelial cell–secreted/anchored ultralarge von Willebrand factor multimeric strings

Complement Component	Mean Intensities ± SD
C3	4186 ± 2452
FB	1675 ± 645
FD	1013 ± 631
FP	913 ± 1067
C5	3128 ± 2087
FH	2262 ± 1385
FI	2581 ± 1710
C4*	31 ± 32

The quantification of AP proteins attached on EC-secreted/anchored ULVWF strings was obtained by immunofluorescent image analysis using monospecific goat polyclonal antibodies to each of the complement components.[2] Methods are described in more detail for C3 and C4 in the legend of **Fig. 3**. The fluorescent intensity at 594 nm from each complement component detected was measured and integrated along the length of the ULVWF string and expressed as intensity per micron of length. There was almost no attachment to the ULVWF strings of C4 (*), an essential component of the classical and lectin complement pathways.

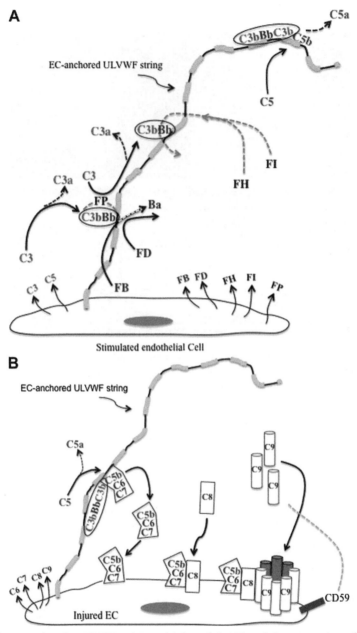

Fig. 4. Cartoons showing ULVWF string activation of the AP and the generation of terminal complement complexes. (*A*) Assembly and activation of the AP on EC-secreted/anchored ULVWF multimeric strings. The binding of AP regulatory proteins, factor H (FH) and factor I (FI), to the ULVWF strings is about one-third less than the binding of C3b (see **Table 1**). Cleavage products C3a and C5a induce histamine release from basophils/mast cells and the chemotaxis of leukocytes. (*B*) Generation of terminal complement complexes after initial AP activation on ULVWF strings. C6 and C7 bind to C5b after C5 is cleaved to C5b by C5 convertase (C3bBbC3b) assembled on the ULVWF multimeric string. The newly formed C5b-7 complex is released from the ULVWF string and can imbed into the membrane of a damaged (or CD59 deficient) EC. The imbedded C5b-7 complex binds a single C8 followed by the attachment of multiple C9 components to produce the pore-forming C5b-9 complex.

also have this effect in vivo. If the secretion/anchorage of ULVWF strings at accelerated rates by stimulated ECs (as during the increased cytokine generation with microbial infection or pregnancy) is associated with a reduced level of ADAMTS-13, then excessive numbers of EC-anchored ULVWF strings will form and persist transiently (ie, at least for a few minutes), leading to prolonged AP activation.[1]

GENERATION OF TERMINAL COMPLEMENT COMPLEXES

In addition to the complement components that participate in initiation and amplification of the AP, HUVECs and other ECs also synthesize the later-acting terminal pathway (TP) components C6, C7, C8, and C9 (see **Fig. 4**B). HUVEC expression of mRNA for each TP component has been detected, although only soluble C7 protein ($\sim$20 ng/10^6 cells) was successfully measured in studies during the early years of this century.[34–36] C7 was also shown not to be primarily synthesized by hepatocytes and not to be an acute phase reactant.[37] ECs may only express and produce low levels of TP (and other complement) components; however, the human vascular system has an immense quantity of ECs ($>10^{13}$ in adults) capable of contributing a considerable portion of each complement protein in circulation.[38]

Active C3 convertase (C3bBb) and C5 convertase (C3bBbC3b) complexes assemble on uncleaved EC-anchored ULVWF strings. C5 convertase generates C5b that can be detected on the ULVWF strings. In our in vitro experiments conducted so far using human ECs,[2] the fluid phase volumes and antibody sensitivities were insufficient to enable the determination if C5b-9 complexes are formed on the EC-anchored ULVWF strings, in the soluble phase, or as complexes inserted into EC membranes. We suspect that C5b molecules generated on the EC-secreted/anchored ULVWF strings combine with soluble C6 and C7 molecules to form C5b-7 complexes that dissociate from the ULVWF strings, escape into the fluid phase, and insert into nearby cell membranes. C8 and multiple C9 molecules may then combine with membrane-imbedded C5b-7 to form C5b-9 complexes. These complexes are even more likely if cells are damaged and deficient in CD59 (which impairs additional C9 molecules from binding to the initial C9 in membrane C5b-9 complexes) (see **Fig. 4**B). Measurement of C5b-9 complexes in the plasma of patients with thrombotic microangiopathies supports the probability that the AP is activated to completion in vivo in ADAMTS-13-deficient TTP, EHEC-HUS, and aHUS.[39,40]

As long as EC-anchored ULVWF strings remain uncleaved, the strings will promote platelet adhesion/aggregation, microvascular thrombosis, and AP assembly-activation. It is likely that cleavage fragments C3a and C5a, both chemotactic and histamine-releasing compounds in an inflammatory response, will be generated (see **Fig. 4**). Possible targets in normal host defense for the lytic C5b-9 complexes generated by activation of the AP on EC secreted/anchored ULVWF strings include potentially harmful microbes or injured/defective cells. C5b-9 complexes inserted into membranes of damaged or defective ECs may also promote the influx of Ca^{2+} and the secretion of additional ULVWF multimeric strings from EC Weibel-Palade bodies,[41] and ULVWF string anchorage, to EC surfaces.

ULTRALARGE VON WILLEBRAND FACTOR MULTIMERS AND ALTERNATIVE COMPLEMENT PATHWAY ACTIVATION IN THE THROMBOTIC MICROANGIOPATHIES
Thrombotic Thrombocytopenic Purpura and Thrombotic Thrombocytopenic Purpura-like Syndromes

Complement activation in vivo in patients with ADAMTS-13-deficient TTP has been reported in several studies. In a report of 23 TTP patients with antibodies to

ADAMTS-13, increased activation of the classical, lectin, and AP was found.[42] In 8 other TTP patients (3 with and 5 without antibodies to ADAMTS-13), there was evidence only for AP activation.[43] Activation of the AP, as determined by elevations of Bb and C5b-9 values in stored plasma samples, was recently found in a retrospective study of 38 patients with acquired ADAMTS-13-deficient TTP.[39]

One adult with autoantibody-induced severe deficiency of ADAMTS-13 and thrombotic microangiopathy unresponsive to plasma exchange recovered following therapy with eculizumab, the humanized monoclonal antibody against C5.[44] The patient was subsequently found to have additional defects in the AP—a polymorphism/mutation in the *CFH* gene (nucleotide 2881G>T, E936D in the FH protein) plus autoantibodies against FH.[18,45] Excessive assembly/activation of AP components on uncleaved EC-secreted/anchored ULVWF strings (because of severe ADAMTS-13 deficiency) may explain this case. It is not yet known if combinations of ADAMTS-13 and AP regulatory defects also account for other TTP-like disorders that are refractory (or only slowly responsive) to plasma exchange-based therapy.

The cause/pathophysiology of TTP-like syndromes in patients who have only mild-modest reductions (eg, to ~25–60% of normal) in plasma ADAMTS-13 is a continuing clinical puzzle. One possible explanation is that some of these patients may have a heterozygous defect of their *ADAMTS13* gene, resulting in modest delay (or inadequate extent) in the cleavage of EC-secreted/anchored ULVWF multimeric strings, likely resulting in some increase in microvascular platelet adhesion/aggregation (**Fig. 2**C) and excessive activation of the AP on any strings that remain uncleaved. This clinical circumstance would be especially threatening if it were to be combined with a polymorphism or heterozygous gene mutation that impairs regulation of the AP (eg, *CFH* or *CFI*).

Enterohemorrhagic Escherichia coli–Hemolytic-Uremic Syndrome

Increased platelet-mediated thrombus formation contributes to the thrombotic microangiopathy and acute renal failure in EHEC-HUS.[1,46–48] These thrombi may be caused, at least partially, by increased secretion or persistence of renal EC-anchored ULVWF strings that induce platelet adherence and aggregation, especially in the glomerular microcirculation.[1,8] Plasma levels of ADAMTS-13 are not severely diminished (to <10%) during EHEC-HUS episodes (see **Fig. 2**C).[3,49–51] There is, however, in human glomerular microvascular endothelial cell and HUVEC in vitro models of EHEC-HUS, a delay in ADAMTS-13-mediated cleavage of EC-secreted/anchored ULVWF multimeric strings under flowing conditions in the presence of nanomolar concentrations of Stx-1 and Stx-2.[8]

Stx-1 binds rapidly to EC-secreted/anchored ULVWF strings—specifically, to A1 and A2 domains of VWF monomers (**Figs. 5** and **6**). This Stx-1 binding decreases the rate of ADAMTS-13-mediated cleavage of the 1605-6 peptide bond in the VWF A2 domain.[52] Stx-1 may bind to regions near the VWF A1-A2 junction and obstruct the access of ADAMTS-13 to the 1605-6 cleavage site in VWF A2 domains. The resulting delay in cleavage of EC-secreted/anchored ULVWF multimeric strings increases modestly the time available for platelet adhesion, activation, and aggregation—and for the binding of C3b and initiation/amplification of the AP. These molecular interactions are likely to be of special pathophysiologic importance during periods of augmented ULVWF string secretion from ECs stimulated by lipopolysaccharide (LPS; endotoxin), Stx-1 and Stx-2,[8,53] and cytokines[1] during an EHEC-HUS episode.

There are additional reports that Stx-2 may bind and inactivate the negative AP regulatory protein, FH,[54] and that endocytosis of the A subunit of Stx-2 may result in reduced mRNA expression and synthesis of CD59, the membrane protein that inhibits

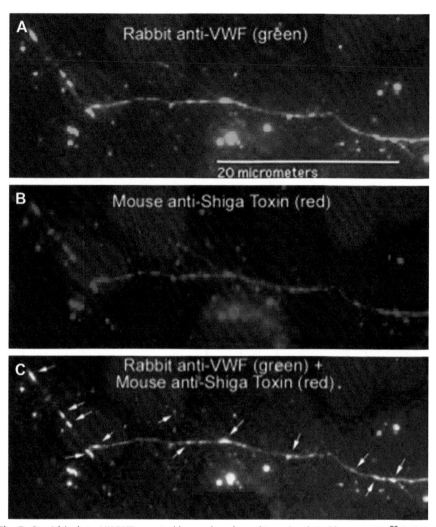

Fig. 5. Stx-1 binds to ULVWF secreted by, and anchored to, stimulated human ECs.[52] HUVECs were stimulated with 100 µM histamine for 2 minutes and then incubated for 15 minutes with rabbit polyclonal antihuman VWF plus chicken antirabbit IgG-AF-488 (*green*) in the presence of 0.1 nM Stx-1. The HUVECs were fixed, washed with phosphate-buffered saline, and stained with mouse monoclonal anti-Stx-1 plus goat antimouse IgG-AF-594 (*red*). (*A*) ULVWF string (*green*); (*B*) Stx-1 (*red*); and (*C*), a combined image of (*A*) and (*B*). The white arrows in (*C*) point to areas on the ULVWF strings with high levels of Stx-1 binding. HUVECs were imaged at ×600 and the cell nuclei were detected with DAPI (*blue*). The Stx-1 attachment on the ULVWF strings was measured as described in the legends for **Table 1** and **Fig. 3**. In control experiments, histamine-stimulated HUVECs were incubated with 0.125-µM cholera toxin (which has structural similarities to Stx-1). The cholera toxin attached to the ULVWF strings in amounts that were 8-fold lower than the Stx-1 binding (data not shown).

the insertion of subsequent C9 molecules into C5b-9 after the initial C9 binds to the TC complex. (This action of CD59 prevents formation of lytic C5b-$[9]_n$ complexes.)[55] FH has also recently been found to reduce *soluble* VWF multimers into smaller forms in vitro,[56] although it is not yet known if the latter is an important antithrombotic function of FH.

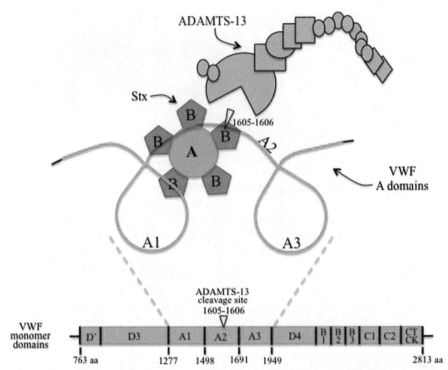

Fig. 6. Cartoon of Stx-1 binding to domains A1 and A2 in the VWF monomeric subunits of EC-anchored ULVWF multimeric strings. Shiga toxin (Stx, 70 kDa) binds to VWF A1 domains (28 kDa) and A2 domains (23 kDa) and restricts ADAMTS-13 (180 kDa) access to its cleavage site within VWF A2 domains. The lower diagram displays the locations of the VWF A1, A2, and A3 domains as well as the ADAMTS-13 cleavage site at amino acids (aa) 1605-1606 of the mature VWF monomer.

Evidence that AP activation occurs in vivo in EHEC-HUS patients has been reported in several studies. Plasma or serum samples in these patients contained depressed values (or cleavage products) of C3, and increased levels of Bb and C5b-9.[50,57–60] Some patients had C3 deposition in the kidneys.[59] Furthermore, the monoclonal antibody, anti-C5 (eculizumab), was used successfully in the treatment of 3 children with severe EHEC-HUS that included neurologic involvement.[60] Eculizumab may also have been therapeutically useful in 8 adults and 1 child with EHEC and extra-renal complications.[9]

Atypical Hemolytic-Uremic Syndrome

Plasma markers for AP overactivation in patients with aHUS were recently reported.[39] These patients had elevations in Bb, C5a, and C5b-9 (all stable during storage). The elevations in C5a and C5b-9 were even higher than in stored plasma samples from patients with acquired ADAMTS-13-deficient TTP.[39]

Patients with aHUS caused by a known AP defect are not inevitably also tested for ADAMTS-13 activity. Some aHUS patients may have a concomitant mild to moderate deficiency of ADAMTS-13 caused by an undetected heterozygous mutation in the *ADAMTS13* gene.[61,62] This undetected heterozygous mutation would be predicted to result in reduction or delay in the cleavage of EC-secreted/anchored ULVWF strings, and to increase the extent of AP activation. One aHUS patient with a gain-of-function *C3* mutation[63] and 3 aHUS patients with loss-of-function *THBD* mutations[64] (causing less effective C3b inactivation by FH and FI) were reported to have "abnormal" ADAMTS-13 activity (amount not specified). A 3-month-old infant at Texas Children's Hospital in Houston, Texas had a severe episode of aHUS in association with a pretransfusion ADAMTS-13 level of 39% and an FH value of 76 µg/mL (normal neonate range is 170–397 µg/mL) (M. Michael, MD, 2011, unpublished). These 5 patients provide clinical examples of AP overactivation in association with diminished (but not absent) ADAMTS-13 activity. If a modest decrease in plasma ADAMTS-13 persists over time (weeks to months) after recovery from an inflammatory episode, this would likely indicate either a heterozygous *ADAMTS13* gene defect or the persistence of a low titer autoantibody against ADAMTS-13.

Individuals with aHUS due to an AP defect are especially prone to develop an episode of aHUS during clinical events associated with the production of inflammatory cytokines (eg, infections, pregnancy).[17] Cytokines (including tumor necrosis factor-α and interleukin-8) initiate EC stimulation and secretion/anchorage of ULVWF multimeric strings.[32] If an aHUS patient were also to have a mild to modest reduction in ADAMTS-13 activity (eg, ~50%), then the EC-anchored ULVWF strings would be expected to persist longer before cleavage, intensify the activation of the already accelerated AP, and promote microvascular platelet adhesion/aggregation.

ULTRALARGE VON WILLEBRAND FACTOR MULTIMERS, ALTERNATIVE COMPLEMENT PATHWAY ACTIVATION, AND THE FORMATION OF SCHISTOCYTES

Intravascular hemolysis and the finding of schistocytes ("cut" red blood cells) on peripheral blood films (ranging from a few to many per oil field) are characteristic of all thrombotic microangiopathies.[65] It has long been presumed that mechanical damage, as occurs as erythrocytes are forced through partially occluded microvessels at high shear rates, is involved in the production of schistocytes. Although mechanical injury may contribute, it is also possible that AP-mediated injury may play a role.

CD59 is a protein tethered to the surfaces of normal RBCs (and other cells) by a glycosyl phosphatidylinositol (GPI)-containing molecule.[66] CD59 inhibits the insertion

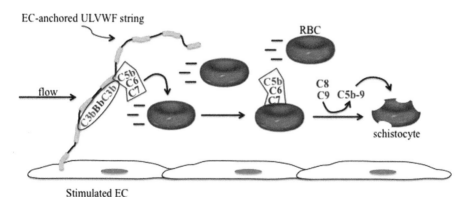

Fig. 7. The cartoon shows a possible mechanism of schistocyte generation by AP activation on EC-secreted/anchored ULVWF strings. Terminal C5b-7 complexes formed on uncleaved EC-anchored ULVWF strings may attach and imbed into the membranes of flowing RBCs. Additional binding of C8 and C9 may then generate lytic C5b-9 complexes in quantities that exceed the regulatory capacity of CD59 on RBC surfaces.

of subsequent C9 molecules into C5b-9 after the initial C9 binds and prevents lytic C5b-9 complex formation.[67] In paroxysmal nocturnal hemoglobinuria (PNH) patients, red cells are defective in CD59 (and in CD55, another GPI-tethered surface molecule that, in contrast to CD59, impairs C3 convertase formation). Schistocytes are found in PNH peripheral blood smears.[68]

In thrombotic microangiopathies, when ECs are stimulated, the EC-secreted/anchored ULVWF multimeric strings may generate terminal complement complexes (TCCs; C5b-9) in quantities that exceed the regulatory capacity of CD59 on otherwise normal RBC surfaces; this would be expected to produce some lysis of RBCs and, possibly, some sublytic injury that may contribute to the formation of schistocytes in the blood of patients with TTP, EHEC-HUS, and aHUS (**Fig. 7**).

SUMMARY

EC-secreted/anchored ULVWF multimeric strings function as activating surfaces for the AP. C3 binds to the EC-secreted/anchored ULVWF strings and promotes the assembly of C3bBb (C3 convertase) and C3bBbC3b (C5 convertase) complexes of the AP. The molecular linkage between inadequately cleaved, EC-secreted/anchored ULVWF multimeric strings and the AP is likely to be of clinical importance in the following: (1) severe ADAMTS-13-deficient TTP, associated predominantly with prolonged persistence of many uncleaved EC-secreted/anchored ULVWF multimeric strings and extensive microvascular platelet adhesion/aggregation (AP activation also occurs); (2) TTP-like syndromes associated with modest ADAMTS-13 deficiency (>10% of normal), persistence of some uncleaved EC-secreted/anchored ULVWF multimeric strings, some microvascular platelet adhesion/aggregation, and some AP activation; (3) EHEC-HUS, associated with Stx/LPS/cytokine-stimulated glomerular EC-secretion/anchorage of ULVWF strings, Stx interference with ADAMTS-13 activity, modestly prolonged persistence of glomerular EC-secreted/anchored ULVWF strings, glomerular platelet adhesion/aggregation, and some AP activation; and (4) precipitation of episodes of aHUS during inflammation (Stx/LPS/cytokine-stimulated EC-secretion/anchorage of ULVWF strings) with extensive overactivation of the abnormal AP on the strings.

REFERENCES

1. Moake JL. Thrombotic microangiopathies. N Engl J Med 2002;347(8):589–600.
2. Turner NA, Moake J. Assembly and activation of alternative complement components on endothelial cell-anchored ultra-large von Willebrand factor links complement and hemostasis-thrombosis. PLoS One 2013;8(3):e59372.
3. Furlan M, Robles R, Galbusera M, et al. von Willebrand factor-cleaving protease in thrombotic thrombocytopenic purpura and the hemolytic-uremic syndrome. N Engl J Med 1998;339(22):1578–84.
4. Furlan M, Robles R, Solenthaler M, et al. Deficient activity of von Willebrand factor-cleaving protease in chronic relapsing thrombotic thrombocytopenic purpura. Blood 1997;89(9):3097–103.
5. Tsai HM, Lian EC. Antibodies to von Willebrand factor-cleaving protease in acute thrombotic thrombocytopenic purpura. N Engl J Med 1998;339(22):1585–94.
6. Garg AX, Suri RS, Barrowman N, et al. Long-term renal prognosis of diarrhea-associated hemolytic uremic syndrome: a systematic review, meta-analysis, and meta-regression. JAMA 2003;290:1360–70.
7. Keir LS, Marks SD, Kim JJ. Shigatoxin-associated hemolytic uremic syndrome: current molecular mechanisms and future therapies. Drug Des Devel Ther 2012;6:195–208.

8. Nolasco LH, Turner NA, Bernardo A, et al. Hemolytic uremic syndrome-associated Shiga toxins promote endothelial-cell secretion and impair ADAMTS13 cleavage of unusually large von Willebrand factor multimers. Blood 2005;106(13):4199–209.

9. Delmas Y, Vendrely B, Clouzeau B, et al. Outbreak of Escherichia coli O104:H4 haemolytic uraemic syndrome in France: outcome with eculizumab. Nephrol Dial Transplant 2014;29(3):565–72.

10. Kielstein JT, Beutel G, Fleig S, et al. Best supportive care and therapeutic plasma exchange with or without eculizumab in Shiga-toxin-producing E. coli O104:H4 induced haemolytic-uraemic syndrome: an analysis of the German STEC-HUS registry. Nephrol Dial Transplant 2012;27(10):3807–15.

11. Cleary TG. Cytotoxin producing Escherichia coli and the hemolytic uremic syndrome. Pediatr Clin North Am 1988;35:485–501.

12. Matussek A, Lauber J, Bergau A, et al. Molecular and functional analysis of Shiga toxin-induced response patterns in human vascular endothelial cells. Blood 2003; 102(4):1323–32.

13. He X, Quinones B, McMahon S, et al. A single-step purification and molecular characterization of functional Shiga toxin 2 variants from pathogenic Escherichia coli. Toxins (Basel) 2012;4(7):487–504.

14. Odumosu O, Nicholas D, Yano H, et al. AB toxins: a paradigm switch from deadly to desirable. Toxins (Basel) 2010;2:1612–45.

15. Tarr PI, Gordon CA, Chandler WL. Shiga-toxin-producing Escherichia coli and haemolytic uraemic syndrome. Lancet 2005;365(9464):1073–86.

16. Trachtman H, Austin C, Lewinski M, et al. Renal and neurological involvement in typical Shiga toxin-associated HUS. Nat Rev Nephrol 2012;8(11):658–69.

17. Loirat C, Frémeaux-Bacchi V. Atypical hemolytic uremic syndrome. Orphanet J Rare Dis 2011;6(1):60.

18. Maga TK, Nishimura CJ, Weaver AE, et al. Mutations in alternative pathway complement proteins in American patients with atypical hemolytic uremic syndrome. Hum Mutat 2010;31(6):E1445–60.

19. Zipfel PF, Edey M, Heinen S, et al. Deletion of complement factor H-related genes CFHR1 and CFHR3 is associated with atypical hemolytic uremic syndrome. PLoS Genet 2007;3(3):e41.

20. Frémeaux-Bacchi V, Miller EC, Liszewski MK, et al. Mutations in complement C3 predispose to development of atypical hemolytic uremic syndrome. Blood 2008; 112(13):4948–52.

21. Goicoechea de Jorge E, Harris CL, Esparza-Gordillo J, et al. Gain-of-function mutations in complement factor B are associated with atypical hemolytic uremic syndrome. Proc Natl Acad Sci U S A 2007;104(1):240–5.

22. Roumenina LT, Loirat C, Dragon-Durey MA, et al. Alternative complement pathway assessment in patients with atypical HUS. J Immunol Methods 2011; 365(1–2):8–26.

23. Law SK, Levine RP. Interaction between the third complement protein and cell surface macromolecules. Proc Natl Acad Sci U S A 1977;74(7):2701–5.

24. Pangburn MK, Ferreira VP, Cortes C. Discrimination between host and pathogens by the complement system. Vaccine 2008;26(Suppl 8):I15–21.

25. Law SK, Dodds AW. The internal thioester and the covalent binding properties of the complement proteins C3 and C4. Protein Sci 1997;6(2):263–74.

26. Schreiber RD, Pangburn MK, Lesavre PH, et al. Initiation of the alternative pathway of complement: recognition of activators by bound C3b and assembly of the entire pathway from six isolated proteins. Proc Natl Acad Sci U S A 1978;75(8):3948–52.

27. Fearon DT, Austen KF, Ruddy S. Formation of a hemolytically active cellular intermediate by the interaction between properdin, factors B and D and the activated third component of complement. J Exp Med 1973;138(6):1305–13.
28. Pillemer L, Blum L, Lepow IH, et al. The properdin system and immunity. I. Demonstration and isolation of a new serum protein, properdin, and its role in immune phenomena. Science 1954;120(3112):279–85.
29. Weiler JM, Daha MR, Austen KF, et al. Control of the amplification convertase of complement by the plasma protein beta1H. Proc Natl Acad Sci U S A 1976;73(9): 3268–72.
30. Kinoshita T, Takata Y, Kozono H, et al. C5 convertase of the alternative complement pathway: covalent linkage between two C3b molecules within the trimolecular complex enzyme. J Immunol 1988;141(11):3895.
31. Rawal N, Pangburn M. Formation of high-affinity C5 convertases of the alternative pathway of complement. J Immunol 2001;166(4):2635–42.
32. Bernardo A, Ball C, Nolasco L, et al. Effects of inflammatory cytokines on the release and cleavage of the endothelial cell-derived ultralarge von Willebrand factor multimers under flow. Blood 2004;104(1):100–6.
33. Huang J, Motto DG, Bundle DR, et al. Shiga toxin B subunits induce VWF secretion by human endothelial cells and thrombotic microangiopathy in ADAMTS13-deficient mice. Blood 2010;116(18):3653–9.
34. Klegeris A, Bissonnette CJ, Dorovini-Zis K, et al. Expression of complement messenger RNAs by human endothelial cells. Brain Res 2000;871(1):1–6.
35. Langeggen H, Berge KE, Macor P, et al. Detection of mRNA for the terminal complement components C5, C6, C8 and C9 in human umbilical vein endothelial cells in vitro. APMIS 2001;109(1):73–8.
36. Langeggen H, Pausa M, Johnson E, et al. The endothelium is an extrahepatic site of synthesis of the seventh component of the complement system. Clin Exp Immunol 2000;121(1):69–76.
37. Wurzner R, Joysey VC, Lachmann PJ. Complement component C7. Assessment of in vivo synthesis after liver transplantation reveals that hepatocytes do not synthesize the majority of human C7. J Immunol 1994;152(9):4624–9.
38. Cines DB, Pollak ES, Buck CA, et al. Endothelial cells in physiology and in the pathophysiology of vascular disorders. Blood 1998;91(10):3527–61.
39. Cataland SR, Holers VM, Geyer S, et al. Biomarkers of the alternative pathway and terminal complement activity at presentation confirms the clinical diagnosis of aHUS and differentiates aHUS from TTP. Blood 2014;123:3733–8.
40. Thurman JM, Marians R, Emlen W, et al. Alternative pathway of complement in children with diarrhea-associated hemolytic uremic syndrome. Clin J Am Soc Nephrol 2009;4(12):1920–4.
41. Hattori R, Hamilton KK, McEver RP, et al. Complement proteins C5b-9 induce secretion of high molecular weight multimers of endothelial von Willebrand factor and translocation of granule membrane protein GMP-140 to the cell surface. J Biol Chem 1989;264(15):9053–60.
42. Reti M, Farkas P, Csuka D, et al. Complement activation in thrombotic thrombocytopenic purpura. J Thromb Haemost 2012;10(5):791–8.
43. Ruiz-Torres MP, Casiraghi F, Galbusera M, et al. Complement activation: the missing link between ADAMTS-13 deficiency and microvascular thrombosis of thrombotic microangiopathies. Thromb Haemost 2005;93(3):443–52.
44. Chapin J, Weksler B, Magro C, et al. Eculizumab in the treatment of refractory idiopathic thrombotic thrombocytopenic purpura. Br J Haematol 2012;157(6): 772–4.

45. Tsai E, Chapin J, Laurence JC, et al. Use of eculizumab in the treatment of a case of refractory, ADAMTS13-deficient thrombotic thrombocytopenic purpura: additional data and clinical follow-up. Br J Haematol 2013;162(4):558–9.
46. Courteciosse V, Habib R, Monnier C. Nonlethal hemolytic and uremic syndromes in children: an electron-microscope study of renal biopsies from six cases. Exp Mol Pathol 1967;7:327–47.
47. Katz J, Krawitz S, Sacks PV, et al. Platelet, erythrocyte, and fibrinogen kinetics in the hemolytic-uremic syndrome of infancy. J Pediatr 1973;83(5):739–48.
48. Siegler RL, Pysher TJ, Tesh VL, et al. Response to single and divided doses of Shiga toxin-1 in a primate model of hemolytic uremic syndrome. J Am Soc Nephrol 2001;12:1458–67.
49. Pysher TJ, Siegler RL, Tesh VL, et al. von Willebrand factor expression in a Shiga toxin-mediated primate model of hemolytic uremic syndrome. Pediatr Dev Pathol 2002;5(5):472–9.
50. Studt JD, Bohm M, Budde U, et al. Measurement of von Willebrand factor-cleaving protease (ADAMTS-13) activity in plasma: a multicenter comparison of different assay methods. J Thromb Haemost 2003;1(9):1882–7.
51. Tsai HM, Chandler WL, Sarode R, et al. von Willebrand factor and von Willebrand factor-cleaving metalloprotease activity in Escherichia coli 0157: H7-associated hemolytic uremic syndrome. Pediatr Res 2001;49:653–9.
52. Lo NC, Turner NA, Cruz MA, et al. Interaction of Shiga toxin with the A-domains and multimers of von Willebrand Factor. J Biol Chem 2013;288(46):33118–23.
53. Morigi M, Galbusera M, Gastoldi S, et al. Alternative pathway activation of complement by Shiga toxin promotes exuberant C3a formation that triggers microvascular thrombosis. J Immunol 2011;187(1):172–80.
54. Orth D, Khan AB, Naim A, et al. Shiga toxin activates complement and binds factor H: evidence for an active role of complement in hemolytic uremic syndrome. J Immunol 2009;182(10):6394–400.
55. Ehrlenbach S, Rosales A, Posch W, et al. Shiga toxin 2 reduces complement inhibitor CD59 expression on human renal tubular epithelial and glomerular endothelial cells. Infect Immun 2013;81(8):2678–85.
56. Nolasco L, Nolasco J, Feng S, et al. Human complement factor H is a reductase for large soluble von Willebrand factor multimers–brief report. Arterioscler Thromb Vasc Biol 2013;33(11):2524–8.
57. Kim Y, Miller K, Michael AF. Breakdown products of C3 and factor B in hemolytic-uremic syndrome. J Lab Clin Med 1977;89(4):845–50.
58. Monnens L, Molenaar J, Lambert PH, et al. The complement system in hemolytic-uremic syndrome in childhood. Clin Nephrol 1980;13(4):168–71.
59. Robson WL, Leung AK, Fick GH, et al. Hypocomplementemia and leukocytosis in diarrhea-associated hemolytic uremic syndrome. Nephron 1992;62(3):296–9.
60. Lapeyraque AL, Malina M, Fremeaux-Bacchi V, et al. Eculizumab in severe Shiga-toxin-associated HUS. N Engl J Med 2011;364(26):2561–3.
61. Feng S, Eyler SJ, Zhang Y, et al. Partial ADAMTS13 deficiency in atypical hemolytic uremic syndrome. Blood 2013;122:1487–93.
62. Feng S, Kroll MH, Nolasco L, et al. Complement activation in thrombotic microangiopathies. Br J Haematol 2013;160(3):404–6.
63. Sartz L, Olin AI, Kristoffersson AC, et al. A novel C3 mutation causing increased formation of the C3 convertase in familial atypical hemolytic uremic syndrome. J Immunol 2012;188(4):2030–7.
64. Delvaeye M, Noris M, De Vriese A, et al. Thrombomodulin mutations in atypical hemolytic-uremic syndrome. N Engl J Med 2009;361(4):345–57.

65. Bull BS, Kuhn IN. The production of schistocytes by fibrin strands (a scanning electron microscope study). Blood 1970;35(1):104–11.
66. Savage WJ, Barber JP, Mukhina GL, et al. Glycosylphosphatidylinositol-anchored protein deficiency confers resistance to apoptosis in PNH. Exp Hematol 2009; 37(1):42–51.
67. Rollins SA, Sims PJ. The complement-inhibitory activity of CD59 resides in its capacity to block incorporation of C9 into membrane C5b-9. J Immunol 1990; 144(9):3478–83.
68. Canalejo K, Riera Cervantes N, Felippo M, et al. Paroxysmal nocturnal haemoglobinuria. Experience over a 10 years period. Int J Lab Hematol 2014;36(2): 213–21.

Shiga Toxin Associated Hemolytic Uremic Syndrome

Lindsay Susan Keir, BSc, MBChB, MRCPCH, PhD[a,b,*]

KEYWORDS

- Thrombotic microangiopathy • Shiga toxin • Complement • Eculizumab

KEY POINTS

- Ninety percent of hemolytic uremic syndrome (HUS) occurs after a gastrointestinal infection with a Shiga toxin (Stx)-producing bacterium, usually *Escherichia coli* O157.
- Stx can directly activate the alternative complement pathway and reduce regulatory protein function.
- Genetic blockade of the alternative pathway is protective in mice, but therapeutic complement blockade in patients has not been consistently beneficial.
- Earlier administration of complement modulatory therapy may be beneficial but a clinical trial is needed to test this hypothesis.
- Further work is needed to define the role of complement in the pathogenesis of Stx HUS and direct therapeutic interventions.

INTRODUCTION

Hemolytic uremic syndrome (HUS) is characterized by the clinical triad of microangiopathic hemolytic anemia, thrombocytopenia, and acute renal injury. It is the leading single cause of pediatric acute kidney injury.[1,2] HUS is a type of thrombotic microangiopathy (TMA).[3] Typically, it occurs after a gastrointestinal infection with a Shiga toxin (Stx)-producing pathogen. This diarrhea- or Stx-associated HUS (D+HUS or Stx-HUS) accounts for 90% of cases.[2] Currently, there are no direct treatments and limited prevention strategies. Most patients recover from the acute illness, but there is a 1% to 4% mortality and one-third of patients are left with long-term medical problems.[2,4] The major challenge facing clinicians and researchers is better understanding the disease pathogenesis in an attempt to develop new therapeutic strategies. With this in

The author has nothing to disclose.
[a] Department of Molecular and Cell Biology, The Scripps Research Institute, MB 216, 10550 North Torrey Pines Road, La Jolla, CA 92037, USA; [b] Academic Renal Unit, University of Bristol, Dorothy Hodgkin Building, Whitson Street, Bristol BS1 3NY, UK
* Department of Molecular and Cell Biology, The Scripps Research Institute, MB 216, 10550 North Torrey Pines Road, La Jolla, CA 92037.
E-mail address: lskeir@doctors.org.uk

Hematol Oncol Clin N Am 29 (2015) 525–539
http://dx.doi.org/10.1016/j.hoc.2015.01.007
0889-8588/15/$ – see front matter © 2015 Elsevier Inc. All rights reserved.

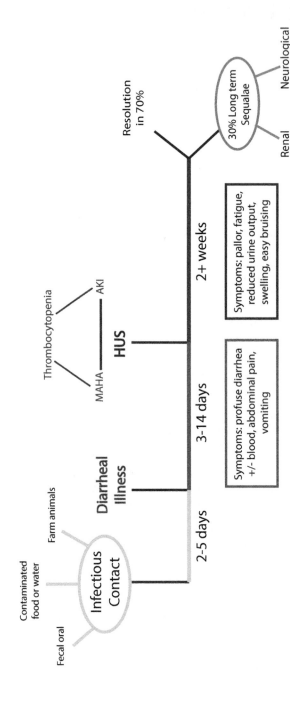

Fig. 1. The timeline of Stx HUS. Stx *E coli* infection is acquired by the fecal oral route from contaminated food or water, ruminant animals (the natural reservoir), or another infected individual. After a 2- to 5-day incubation period, profuse diarrhea develops that can be bloody. Vomiting and abdominal pain can also occur. Three to 14 days later, features of HUS arise. Symptoms can be vague with pallor, lethargy, reduced urine output, swelling and easy bruising. The clinical triad of microangiopathic hemolytic anemia (MAHA), thrombocytopenia, and acute kidney injury (AKI) characterize HUS. Disease duration can vary with some patients recovering over several weeks. Others can take longer. Most will make a full recovery from HUS, but 30% will have long-standing renal or neurologic impairment.

mind, attention has turned to advances in the understanding of a related condition, complement-mediated HUS. This atypical HUS subtype is now successfully treated with the C5 monoclonal antibody, eculizumab.[5] Its success prompted clinicians to ask if it could also be used to treat Stx HUS and for researchers to examine the role of complement in the pathogenesis of this disease.

EPIDEMIOLOGY

Worldwide, Stx-producing *Escherichia coli* causes 2.8 million illnesses annually.[6] In the United States, it causes more than 265,000 illnesses per year[7] with 3600 hospitalizations and 30 deaths.[7] The global incidence of Stx HUS is 0.2 to 4.28 people per 100,000 population.[8] Seasonal variation occurs with more cases in summer.[9] Stx HUS is more common in children, particularly those under the age of 5.[10] *E coli* O157, the most common Stx-producing *E coli*, is responsible for 724 hospitalizations and 11 deaths per year in this age group in the United States.[11]

CLINICAL COURSE

Patients infected with a Stx-producing pathogen usually develop a profuse diarrheal illness 2 to 5 days later (**Fig. 1**).[10] Signs and symptoms of HUS occur after the diarrhea, but only in 10% to 15% of people infected with *E coli* O157.[1,10] The risk of developing Stx HUS is influenced by the organisms serotype,[10] as illustrated in the *E coli* O104 outbreak, where 22% of infected patients developed HUS.[12] Host factors also play a role (**Box 1**).[12,13]

Signs and Symptoms

Symptoms of HUS can be vague (see **Fig. 1**). Medical examination reveals signs of oligoanuric kidney injury with fluid overload and hypertension. There is a disease spectrum. More severely affected patients may show signs of other organ involvement, particularly cerebral, pancreatic, hepatic, and cardiac.[10,14,15]

PATHOLOGY

The pathologic feature of HUS is TMA. This term describes characteristic endothelial cell damage (**Fig. 2A**),[16] which leads to complete or partial vessel obstruction, resulting in fragmented red blood cells. Characteristic laboratory findings include consumptive thrombocytopenia and microangiopathic hemolytic anemia.[16,17] Organ ischemia occurs with symptoms determined by the vascular bed affected. In glomerular TMA,

---

Box 1
Host factors that increase the risk of developing Shiga toxin-associated hemolytic uremic syndrome

Host factors that increase risk of HUS

Extremes of age (<5 y,[13] >75 y[12])

Vomiting[12]

>3 days of diarrhea[13]

Blood in stool[12]

High white cell count (>13,000/μL)[13]

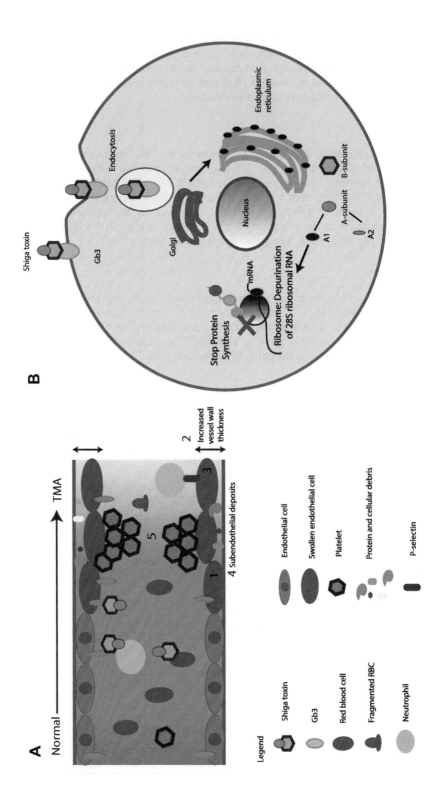

there will be evidence of renal impairment, but if TMA affects the brain neurologic symptoms develop.[16,18]

PATHOGENESIS

Stx-producing bacteria infect the large intestine causing colitis.[19] The toxin produced crosses the gastrointestinal epithelium and enters the circulation possibly via globote-traosylceramide (Gb4) cellular receptors,[20] but monocytes[21] and neutrophils[22] may also be involved. Stx targets cells that express globotriosylceramide (Gb3) receptors. Free Stx has never been detected in patient blood.[23] Erythrocytes, neutrophils, and platelets[24–26] have been implicated in Stx carriage,[19,27] but this may not be via Gb3 receptors.[24] Recently, it was reported that neutrophils bind Stx via toll-like receptor 4 (TLR4).[28] It is hypothesized that TLR4 has a lower affinity for Stx than Gb3, so when Stx arrives at a Gb3 expressing organ, such as the kidney, it preferentially detaches from the circulating cells and binds to the Gb3-expressing cells.

Cellular Effects

When Stx binds cellular Gb3, the toxin is internalized by endocytosis and, if expressed in a detergent-resistant membrane, undergoes retrograde transport to the endoplasmic reticulum (see **Fig. 2**B).[29,30] Ultimately, Stx stops cellular protein synthesis (see **Fig. 2**B) and causes apoptosis with damage to the integrity of the endothelium and exposure of the subendothelial layer leading to TMA.[16,18,21,31,32] Stx may have other effects, including increasing synthesis of pro-inflammatory cytokines,[33] directly damaging DNA,[21,34] generating microparticles,[35,36] causing impaired cellular oxidative balance,[37–39] and interacting with complement proteins.

THE COMPLEMENT SYSTEM IN SHIGA TOXIN-ASSOCIATED HEMOLYTIC UREMIC SYNDROME PATHOGENESIS
Clinical Evidence of Complement Activation in Shiga Toxin-Associated Hemolytic Uremic Syndrome

Complement activation occurs in Stx HUS patients (**Box 2**).[40–43] It may be an early disease feature because activated factor B (Bb) fragments and soluble membrane attack complex (MAC) were detected in patient plasma at the time of hospital admission before starting treatment.[43] One month later, levels had normalized.[43] Platelet-leukocyte complexes and microparticles with evidence of complement activation on

----

Fig. 2. Stx pathogenesis. (*A*) The pathologic feature of HUS is TMA, which describes features of endothelial cell damage, including (*1*) endotheliosis, (*2*) increased vessel wall thickness, (*3*) detachment of cells from the basement membrane, with (*4*) accumulation of protein and cellular debris in the subendothelial space.[16,18,31] A procoagulant, activated endothelial phenotype develops with expression of von Willebrand factor attracting platelets and inducing formation of intraluminal microthrombi (*5*). P-selectin expression attracts neutrophils to the site. Stx carried by blood cells causes TMA by binding to Gb3 receptors on the endothelial cells. (*B*) Stx binds to Gb3 cell surface receptors. The Stx-receptor complex is internalized by endocytosis and undergoes retrograde transport to the endoplasmic reticulum via the Golgi stack. In the endoplasmic reticulum, Stx is split into 2: the α and β subunits. The α subunit mimics a misfolded protein and, using the hosts own machinery, is translocated to the cytosol. Here, the enzymatically active A1 fragment (27.5 kDa) causes depurination of adenosine at a highly conserved loop of 28S ribosomal RNA of the 60S ribosomal subunit, stopping protein synthesis and activating the ribosomal stress response.

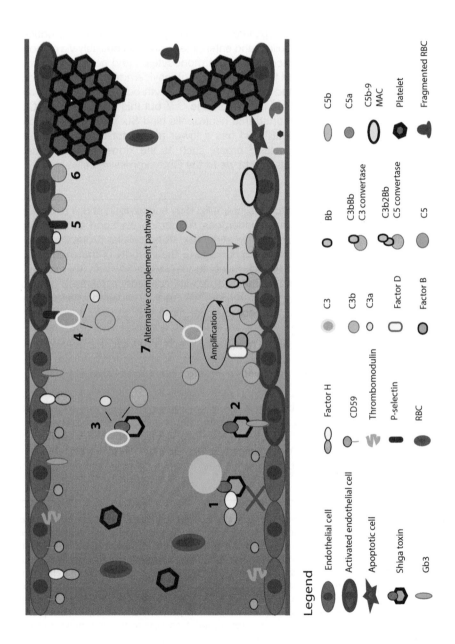

Legend

Endothelial cell	Factor H	C3	Bb	C5b
Activated endothelial cell	CD59	C3b	C3bBb C3 convertase	C5a
Apoptotic cell	Thrombomodulin	C3a	C3b2Bb C5 convertase	C5b-9 MAC
Shiga toxin	P-selectin	Factor D	C5	Platelet
Gb3	RBC	Factor B		Fragmented RBC

7 Alternative complement pathway

Amplification

Box 2
Evidence of complement activation in Shiga toxin-associated hemolytic uremic syndrome patients

Low serum C3[16]

C3 breakdown fragments (C3b, C3c, and C3d)[17–19]

Factor B breakdown fragments (Bb)[17–19]

Serum-soluble MAC[19]

C3 deposits in kidney[16]

C3/C9 covered platelet-leukocyte complexes and microparticles[20]

---

their surface have also been identified.[35] These clinical observations show that complement is activated in Stx HUS but not how it contributes to disease pathogenesis.

In Vitro Evidence

Shiga toxin inhibits protective complement regulators
Stx can bind to and inhibit the complement regulatory function of complement factor H (CFH)[44] and CFH-related protein 1,[45] which may make cells vulnerable to complement-mediated damage (**Fig. 3**). Stx targets the membrane-binding portions of CFH, so although it can still regulate complement in fluid phase, it cannot on the cell surface. This phenomena is the same as that produced by the CFH loss-of-function mutations associated with atypical, complement-mediated HUS.[46] Furthermore, glomerular endothelial cell expression of the membrane-bound complement regulator CD59[47] and the complement and coagulation regulator thrombomodulin (TM)[48] were reduced by Stx. TM loss may be due to increased cellular shedding,[49] which could explain the high serum TM levels found in Stx HUS patients.[50]

Shiga toxin activates complement
Stx can directly activate complement predominately via the alternative pathway (see **Fig. 3**).[44] Endothelial cells pretreated with Stx and exposed to human serum expressed P-selectin can bind and activate C3 (see **Fig. 3**).[49] The formation of C3a further enhances P-selectin expression, decreases TM expression, and thrombosis ensues.[49] In vitro, C3 complement deposits occurred before thrombin deposition, suggesting that complement deposition could trigger thrombosis. Inhibiting complement activation abolished these effects.

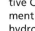

Fig. 3. The role of complement in Stx HUS pathogenesis. Stx can bind to and inhibit protective CFH (*1*) and reduces expression of CD59 and TM (*2*). It can also directly activate complement via the alternative pathway via interactions with C3 (*3*). Endothelial cell P-selectin also hydrolyses C3 to C3a and C3b (*4*). The anaphylatoxin C3a enhances P-selectin expression and reduces TM (*5*). C3 deposits occur on the endothelium leading to activation of the alternative pathway before thrombin is seen (*6*). The alternative pathway is illustrated (*7*). C3b combines with the Bb fragment of factor B to form the C3 convertase, C3bBb. This is mediated by factor D. The C3 convertase causes an amplification loop hydrolyzing C3 to produce more C3b, combining with the C3 convertase to form a C5 convertase (C3b2Bb); this hydrolyses C5 to C5a (anaphylatoxin) and C5b, which combines with C6-C9 to form the MAC. Cell lysis occurs, exposing the subendothelial matrix. Inflammation caused by the anaphylatoxins activates endothelial cells, leading to a procoagulant phenotype with von Willebrand factor expression. Activation of the complement system is known to active the coagulation system also, leading to the development of TMA. RBC, red blood cell.

MOUSE MODELS

Murine models of Stx HUS are used to study the disease but do not precisely replicate human pathology because mice lack glomerular Gb3 receptors.[51] Instead, they develop renal tubular damage. Heterozygous CFH-deficient mice[52] and C5-deficient mice[53] developed the same tubular damage as wild-type mice, suggesting complement does not play a role in this murine model. Mice treated with higher doses of Stx and lipopolysaccharide (LPS) do develop some intraglomerular platelet clumps and endothelial swelling; this is the best published Stx HUS model to date.[54] In this model, mice have reduced glomerular TM expression with C3 and C9 glomerular deposits, suggesting complement activation. Mice lacking the TM complement regulatory (lectin) domain had a more severe clinical phenotype when challenged with Stx and LPS.[55] Similarly challenged factor B knockout mice showed no C3 deposits and less thrombocytopenia, and renal function was maintained.[49] In this murine model of Stx HUS, alternative pathway blockade through genetic knockout was protective. Further studies suggested a role for complement activation specifically in the specialized glomerular epithelial cell, the podocyte,[56] highlighting that Stx has effects on other cell types too. Further work is needed to confirm these findings in patients.

TREATMENT

There is no direct treatment for Stx HUS. Medical management is supportive, focusing on stabilizing the patient until natural disease resolution occurs and recovery begins.[4,57] Most patients will be treated symptomatically with careful fluid and electrolyte management, nutritional support, and medication for hypertension.[1,10] More severely affected patients require renal replacement therapy[15] and may need intensive care. A systematic review reported that all therapies tested to date showed no benefit over best supportive care (BSC).[58] Given the evidence that complement may be dysregulated, therapies that modulate this system have been used but with conflicting results.

Modulating Complement to Treat Shiga Toxin-Associated Hemolytic Uremic Syndrome

Plasma exchange
Plasma exchange is sometimes used in severe Stx HUS with neurologic symptoms despite a lack of evidence. This practice is more common in adults wherein thrombotic thrombocytopenic purpura is considered in the differential. The rationale for use goes beyond modulating the complement system and may also relate to removing antibodies, proinflammatory, and procoagulant factors. Two multicenter randomized controlled trials were performed in the 1980s. One reported no benefit with plasma infusion over BSC,[59] while the other suggested modest benefit 1 and 6 months after acute illness but no difference at 1 year.[60] It is important to note that these trials were carried out before routine testing for Stx E coli and so the patient group may be heterogeneous. More recently, a long-term surveillance study found plasma exchange was significantly associated with poor long-term outcomes, even when accounting for its use in the most severe cases,[4] contrasting the beneficial effects reported in atypical, complement-mediated HUS.[31,61] The use of plasma exchange was advocated by the German Nephrology Society during the 2011 outbreak,[62] but no patient benefit resulted from its use alone or with steroids in adults or children.[63,64] One Danish group suggested early use may ameliorate the disease course, but only 5 patients were studied.[65] Therefore, evidence is lacking to support the use of plasma exchange in this disease.

Therapeutic complement blockade
Complement blockade is being used in Stx HUS by administering the C5 monoclonal antibody, eculizumab, despite a lack of consistent evidence on benefit and significant economic implications.

E coli O157

Three severely affected children with *E coli* O157 were the first to receive eculizumab because of severe neurologic symptoms.[66] It was given relatively late in the disease. They had evidence of complement activation in blood samples. All 3 patients recovered with resolution of neurologic symptoms 7 to 12 days after complement blockade. Benefit was attributed to eculizumab. Two patients had also received plasma exchange, and all had received other supportive measures before complement blockade. It must be remembered that 70% of all Stx HUS patients recover with time and supportive therapy alone.[4,57] It is unclear from this study whether the improvements seen were different to natural recovery even in the setting of severe disease.

E coli O104

Adults
The second evaluation of eculizumab in Stx HUS was during the 2011 *E coli* O104 outbreak.[62,64,67–70] This outbreak was not typical of Stx HUS because 68% of patients affected were adult women, and there were higher rates of severe disease with neurologic involvement.[68,69] Several groups reported using eculizumab in this outbreak, but most report no benefit over standard care.[63,68,69] In most cases, eculizumab was administered after supportive therapy and usually after plasma exchange; this was always several days into hospital admission and eculizumab was given to only the most severely affected. Patients were not randomized, and there was no adequate control group. One group did compare BSC with plasma exchange plus or minus eculizumab in adult patients[68]; however, these patients were not randomized and there were significant differences between groups. For example, some BSC patients had advanced directives and refused dialysis.[68] For this reason, there was greater mortality in the BSC group but lower median hospital stays and creatinine at discharge. In contrast, a French group used eculizumab earlier within 0 to 4 days of HUS caused by *E coli* O104 HUS.[71] The group studied 9 patients. Six had not received prior plasma therapy. All had extrarenal complications. Within 3 days, platelet counts increased. The authors attribute this to early use of eculizumab.

Pediatric perspective
Pediatric data were collected for 90 children from 13 German centers.[64] Most patients received BSC only; however, 19% received plasma exchange, and 13 patients received eculizumab. Four patients received only BSC before complement blockade,

Table 1
Percentage of patients with long-term complications 5 years after acute Shiga toxin-associated hemolytic uremic syndrome

Chronic Health Problem	% Affected 5 y After Acute Disease
Proteinuria[70,71]	19
Hypertension[70,71]	9
Chronic kidney disease/↓ GFR[70,71]	7
Neurologic problems[4]	4

Abbraviation: GFR, glomerular filtration rate.

Box 3
Poor prognostic indicators
Factor associated with poor prognosis
Oliguria persisting >4 wk[70]
Acute dialysis greater than 15 d[4]
Neurologic symptoms[14]
Plasma therapy[4]
High white cell count[4]

while the rest also had plasma exchange. Three patients received protein C. Across all treatment groups, 1 patient died, 4.4% were left with chronic kidney disease, and 22% had ongoing neurologic problems. These rates are comparable to previously reported cases.[4,10,14,57] Specific outcomes for the different treatment groups were not reported because of small numbers. However, the authors conclude that, based on their experience, plasma exchange and eculizumab showed no short-term benefit.

Summary
Ultimately, no benefit could be attributed to the use of eculizumab in patients treated during this outbreak.[63,64,68] So far, most patients received eculizumab late in the disease course and after other therapeutic interventions. However, there are data suggesting that complement activation occurs early in the disease process.[43,49] Therefore, administering eculizumab earlier may be more effective at modifying the disease pathogenesis and have a greater influence on patient outcome, possibly explaining the positive results from Delmas and colleagues.[71] A randomized controlled trial is needed to address this issue.

PROGNOSIS

Although 70% of Stx HUS patients make a full recovery, 1% to 4% of Stx HUS cases are fatal.[2,57,72] Disease severity and clinical course impact prognosis. Those with mild disease gradually improve with recovery of renal function over a few weeks.[4,57,73] Severe disease can take longer. Approximately 30% of patients are left with long-term problems.[57] Commonly, this affects the kidneys, but persistent neurologic sequelae also occur (**Table 1**).[4,73,74] Most long-term problems persist from the acute illness, but some patients who seem to initially recover from the acute illness can develop proteinuria and hypertension 1 to 2 years later.[4] Therefore, patients with Stx HUS should be followed up for years after the acute illness. Factors associated with a poor prognosis are listed in **Box 3**.[4,14,73]

SUMMARY

The TMA Stx HUS typically occurs after diarrheal infection with a Stx-producing *E coli*. It carries significant morbidity and mortality, but there are no effective treatments. Most patients recover with supportive care, but 30% have long-term sequelae. Therefore, all patients should be followed up after acute illness. Complement is activated in this disease, but its role in disease pathogenesis is not completely defined. There is a critical need to understand this better because complement blockade is being used in patients despite the lack of robust evidence. This may expose patients to unnecessary drug treatment with potential side effects and has financial implications because eculizumab is an expensive drug.[75] If complement plays a role in Stx HUS and complement modulatory therapy is to be used, the optimal timing of administration and duration of treatment must be determined. Current evidence suggests that early use may be indicated. The treatment course is likely to be short given the acute nature of the disease and so costs would be less than those associated with chronic diseases such as atypical HUS and paroxysmal nocturnal hemoglobinuria. A randomized controlled trial would help address these issues and guide therapeutic practice.

REFERENCES

1. Ake JA, Jelacic S, Ciol MA, et al. Relative nephroprotection during Escherichia coli O157:H7 infections: association with intravenous volume expansion. Pediatrics 2005;115(6):e673–80.
2. Bitzan M. Treatment options for HUS secondary to Escherichia coli O157:H7. Kidney Int Suppl 2009;(112):S62–6.
3. Siegler RL. The hemolytic uremic syndrome. Pediatr Clin North Am 1995;42(6): 1505–29.
4. Rosales A, Hofer J, Zimmerhackl LB, et al. Need for long-term follow-up in enterohemorrhagic Escherichia coli-associated hemolytic uremic syndrome due to late-emerging sequelae. Clin Infect Dis 2012;54(10):1413–21.
5. Gruppo RA, Rother RP. Eculizumab for congenital atypical hemolytic-uremic syndrome. N Engl J Med 2009;360(5):544–6.
6. Majowicz SE, Scallan E, Jones-Bitton A, et al. Global incidence of human Shiga toxin-producing Escherichia coli infections and deaths: a systematic review and knowledge synthesis. Foodborne Pathog Dis 2014;11(6):447–55.
7. Scallan E, Griffin PM, Angulo FJ, et al. Foodborne illness acquired in the United States–unspecified agents. Emerg Infect Dis 2011;17(1):16–22.
8. Serna A, Boedeker EC. Pathogenesis and treatment of Shiga toxin-producing Escherichia coli infections. Curr Opin Gastroenterol 2008;24(1):38–47.
9. Money P, Kelly AF, Gould SW, et al. Cattle, weather and water: mapping Escherichia coli O157:H7 infections in humans in England and Scotland. Environ Microbiol 2010;12(10):2633–44.
10. Scheiring J, Andreoli SP, Zimmerhackl LB. Treatment and outcome of Shiga-toxin-associated hemolytic uremic syndrome (HUS). Pediatr Nephrol 2008;23(10): 1749–60.
11. Scallan E, Mahon BE, Hoekstra RM, et al. Estimates of illnesses, hospitalizations and deaths caused by major bacterial enteric pathogens in young children in the United States. Pediatr Infect Dis J 2013;32(3):217–21.
12. Zoufaly A, Cramer JP, Vettorazzi E, et al. Risk factors for development of hemolytic uremic syndrome in a cohort of adult patients with STEC 0104:H4 infection. PLoS One 2013;8(3):e59209.
13. Tserenpuntsag B, Chang HG, Smith PF, et al. Hemolytic uremic syndrome risk and Escherichia coli O157:H7. Emerg Infect Dis 2005;11(12):1955–7.
14. Nathanson S, Kwon T, Elmaleh M, et al. Acute neurological involvement in diarrhea-associated hemolytic uremic syndrome. Clin J Am Soc Nephrol 2010; 5(7):1218–28.
15. Gianviti A, Tozzi AE, De Petris L, et al. Risk factors for poor renal prognosis in children with hemolytic uremic syndrome. Pediatr Nephrol 2003;18(12):1229–35.
16. Ruggenenti P, Noris M, Remuzzi G. Thrombotic microangiopathy, hemolytic uremic syndrome, and thrombotic thrombocytopenic purpura. Kidney Int 2001; 60(3):831–46.

17. Zheng XL, Sadler JE. Pathogenesis of thrombotic microangiopathies. Annu Rev Pathol 2008;3:249–77.
18. Barbour T, Johnson S, Cohney S, et al. Thrombotic microangiopathy and associated renal disorders. Nephrol Dial Transplant 2012;27(7):2673–85.
19. Zoja C, Buelli S, Morigi M. Shiga toxin-associated hemolytic uremic syndrome: pathophysiology of endothelial dysfunction. Pediatr Nephrol 2010;25(11): 2231–40.
20. Zumbrun SD, Hanson L, Sinclair JF, et al. Human intestinal tissue and cultured colonic cells contain globotriaosylceramide synthase mRNA and the alternate Shiga toxin receptor globotetraosylceramide. Infect Immun 2010;78(11): 4488–99.
21. Bauwens A, Betz J, Meisen I, et al. Facing glycosphingolipid-Shiga toxin interaction: dire straits for endothelial cells of the human vasculature. Cell Mol Life Sci 2013;70(3):425–57.
22. Hurley BP, Thorpe CM, Acheson DW. Shiga toxin translocation across intestinal epithelial cells is enhanced by neutrophil transmigration. Infect Immun 2001; 69(10):6148–55.
23. Brigotti M, Tazzari PL, Ravanelli E, et al. Clinical relevance of shiga toxin concentrations in the blood of patients with hemolytic uremic syndrome. Pediatr Infect Dis J 2011;30(6):486–90.
24. Griener TP, Mulvey GL, Marcato P, et al. Differential binding of Shiga toxin 2 to human and murine neutrophils. J Med Microbiol 2007;56(Pt 11):1423–30.
25. Ghosh SA, Polanowska-Grabowska RK, Fujii J, et al. Shiga toxin binds to activated platelets. J Thromb Haemost 2004;2(3):499–506.
26. Bitzan M, Richardson S, Huang C, et al. Evidence that verotoxins (Shiga-like toxins) from Escherichia coli bind to P blood group antigens of human erythrocytes in vitro. Infect Immun 1994;62(8):3337–47.
27. Schüller S. Shiga toxin interaction with human intestinal epithelium. Toxins (Basel) 2011;3(6):626–39.
28. Brigotti M, Carnicelli D, Arfilli V, et al. Identification of TLR4 as the receptor that recognizes Shiga toxins in human neutrophils. J Immunol 2013;191(9): 4748–58.
29. Johannes L, Römer W. Shiga toxins–from cell biology to biomedical applications. Nat Rev Microbiol 2010;8(2):105–16.
30. Spooner RA, Lord JM. How ricin and Shiga toxin reach the cytosol of target cells: retrotranslocation from the endoplasmic reticulum. Curr Top Microbiol Immunol 2012;357:19–40.
31. Clark WF. Thrombotic microangiopathy: current knowledge and outcomes with plasma exchange. Semin Dial 2012;25(2):214–9.
32. Huang J, Motto DG, Bundle DR, et al. Shiga toxin B subunits induce VWF secretion by human endothelial cells and thrombotic microangiopathy in ADAMTS13-deficient mice. Blood 2010;116(18):3653–9.
33. Thorpe CM, Hurley BP, Lincicome LL, et al. Shiga toxins stimulate secretion of interleukin-8 from intestinal epithelial cells. Infect Immun 1999;67(11):5985–93.
34. Brigotti M, Alfieri R, Sestili P, et al. Damage to nuclear DNA induced by Shiga toxin 1 and ricin in human endothelial cells. FASEB J 2002;16(3):365–72.
35. Ståhl AL, Sartz L, Karpman D. Complement activation on platelet-leukocyte complexes and microparticles in enterohemorrhagic Escherichia coli-induced hemolytic uremic syndrome. Blood 2011;117(20):5503–13.
36. Ge S, Hertel B, Emden SH, et al. Microparticle generation and leucocyte death in Shiga toxin-mediated HUS. Nephrol Dial Transplant 2012;27(7):2768–75.

37. Aiassa V, Baronetti JL, Paez PL, et al. Increased advanced oxidation of protein products and enhanced total antioxidant capacity in plasma by action of toxins of Escherichia coli STEC. Toxicol In Vitro 2011;25(1):426–31.

38. Gomez SA, Abrey-Recalde MJ, Panek CA, et al. The oxidative stress induced in vivo by shiga toxin-2 contributes to the pathogenicity of haemolytic uraemic syndrome. Clin Exp Immunol 2013;173(3):463–72.

39. Dran GI, Fernández GC, Rubel CJ, et al. Protective role of nitric oxide in mice with Shiga toxin-induced hemolytic uremic syndrome. Kidney Int 2002;62(4):1338–48.

40. Robson WL, Leung AK, Fick GH, et al. Hypocomplementemia and leukocytosis in diarrhea-associated hemolytic uremic syndrome. Nephron 1992;62(3):296–9.

41. Monnens L, Molenaar J, Lambert PH, et al. The complement system in hemolytic-uremic syndrome in childhood. Clin Nephrol 1980;13(4):168–71.

42. Kim Y, Miller K, Michael AF. Breakdown products of C3 and factor B in hemolytic-uremic syndrome. J Lab Clin Med 1977;89(4):845–50.

43. Thurman JM, Marians R, Emlen W, et al. Alternative pathway of complement in children with diarrhea-associated hemolytic uremic syndrome. Clin J Am Soc Nephrol 2009;4(12):1920–4.

44. Orth D, Khan AB, Naim A, et al. Shiga toxin activates complement and binds factor H: evidence for an active role of complement in hemolytic uremic syndrome. J Immunol 2009;182(10):6394–400.

45. Poolpol K, Orth-Höller D, Speth C, et al. Interaction of Shiga toxin 2 with complement regulators of the factor H protein family. Mol Immunol 2014;58(1):77–84.

46. Pickering MC, de Jorge EG, Martinez-Barricarte R, et al. Spontaneous hemolytic uremic syndrome triggered by complement factor H lacking surface recognition domains. J Exp Med 2007;204(6):1249–56.

47. Ehrlenbach S, Rosales A, Posch W, et al. Shiga toxin 2 reduces complement inhibitor CD59 expression on human renal tubular epithelial and glomerular endothelial cells. Infect Immun 2013;81(8):2678–85.

48. Fernández GC, Te Loo MW, van der Velden TJ, et al. Decrease of thrombomodulin contributes to the procoagulant state of endothelium in hemolytic uremic syndrome. Pediatr Nephrol 2003;18(10):1066–8.

49. Morigi M, Galbusera M, Gastoldi S, et al. Alternative pathway activation of complement by Shiga toxin promotes exuberant C3a formation that triggers microvascular thrombosis. J Immunol 2011;187(1):172–80.

50. Nevard CH, Blann AD, Jurd KM, et al. Markers of endothelial cell activation and injury in childhood haemolytic uraemic syndrome. Pediatr Nephrol 1999;13(6):487–92.

51. Rutjes NW, Binnington BA, Smith CR, et al. Differential tissue targeting and pathogenesis of verotoxins 1 and 2 in the mouse animal model. Kidney Int 2002;62(3):832–45.

52. Paixão-Cavalcante D, Botto M, Cook HT, et al. Shiga toxin-2 results in renal tubular injury but not thrombotic microangiopathy in heterozygous factor H-deficient mice. Clin Exp Immunol 2009;155(2):339–47.

53. Barrett TJ, Potter ME, Strockbine NA. Evidence for participation of the macrophage in Shiga-like toxin II-induced lethality in mice. Microb Pathog 1990;9(2):95–103.

54. Keepers TR, Psotka MA, Gross LK, et al. A murine model of HUS: Shiga toxin with lipopolysaccharide mimics the renal damage and physiologic response of human disease. J Am Soc Nephrol 2006;17(12):3404–14.

55. Zoja C, Locatelli M, Pagani C, et al. Lack of the lectin-like domain of thrombomodulin worsens Shiga toxin-associated hemolytic uremic syndrome in mice. J Immunol 2012;189(7):3661–8.

56. Locatelli M, Buelli S, Pezzotta A, et al. Shiga toxin promotes podocyte injury in experimental hemolytic uremic syndrome via activation of the alternative pathway of complement. J Am Soc Nephrol 2014;25(8):1786–98.
57. Spinale JM, Ruebner RL, Copelovitch L, et al. Long-term outcomes of Shiga toxin hemolytic uremic syndrome. Pediatr Nephrol 2013;28(11):2097–105.
58. Michael M, Elliott EJ, Craig JC, et al. Interventions for hemolytic uremic syndrome and thrombotic thrombocytopenic purpura: a systematic review of randomized controlled trials. Am J Kidney Dis 2009;53(2):259–72.
59. Rizzoni G, Claris-Appiani A, Edefonti A, et al. Plasma infusion for hemolytic-uremic syndrome in children: results of a multicenter controlled trial. J Pediatr 1988;112(2):284–90.
60. Loirat C, Sonsino E, Hinglais N, et al. Treatment of the childhood haemolytic uraemic syndrome with plasma. A multicentre randomized controlled trial. The French Society of Paediatric Nephrology. Pediatr Nephrol 1988;2(3): 279–85.
61. Noris M, Remuzzi G. Atypical hemolytic uremic syndrome. N Engl J Med 2009; 361:1676–87.
62. Kemper MJ. Outbreak of hemolytic uremic syndrome caused by E. coli O104:H4 in Germany: a pediatric perspective. Pediatr Nephrol 2012;27(2):161–4.
63. Menne J, Nitschke M, Stingele R, et al. Validation of treatment strategies for enterohaemorrhagic Escherichia coli O104:H4 induced haemolytic uraemic syndrome: case-control study. BMJ 2012;345:e4565.
64. Loos S, Ahlenstiel T, Kranz B, et al. An outbreak of Shiga toxin-producing Escherichia coli O104:H4 hemolytic uremic syndrome in Germany: presentation and short-term outcome in children. Clin Infect Dis 2012;55(6):753–9.
65. Colic E, Dieperink H, Titlestad K, et al. Management of an acute outbreak of diarrhoea-associated haemolytic uraemic syndrome with early plasma exchange in adults from southern Denmark: an observational study. Lancet 2011;378(9796): 1089–93.
66. Lapeyraque AL, Malina M, Fremeaux-Bacchi V, et al. Eculizumab in severe Shiga-toxin-associated HUS. N Engl J Med 2011;364(26):2561–3.
67. Greinacher A, Friesecke S, Abel P, et al. Treatment of severe neurological deficits with IgG depletion through immunoadsorption in patients with Escherichia coli O104:H4-associated haemolytic uraemic syndrome: a prospective trial. Lancet 2011;378(9797):1166–73.
68. Kielstein JT, Beutel G, Fleig S, et al. Best supportive care and therapeutic plasma exchange with or without eculizumab in Shiga-toxin-producing E. coli O104:H4 induced haemolytic-uraemic syndrome: an analysis of the German STEC-HUS registry. Nephrol Dial Transplant 2012;27(10):3807–15.
69. Menne J, Kielstein JT, Wenzel U, et al. Treatment of typical hemolytic-uremic syndrome: knowledge gained from analyses of the 2011 E. coli outbreak. Internist (Berl) 2012;53(12):1420–30 [in German].
70. Nitschke M, Sayk F, Härtel C, et al. Association between azithromycin therapy and duration of bacterial shedding among patients with Shiga toxin-producing enteroaggregative Escherichia coli O104:H4. JAMA 2012; 307(10):1046–52.
71. Delmas Y, Vendrely B, Clouzeau B, et al. Outbreak of Escherichia coli O104:H4 haemolytic uraemic syndrome in France: outcome with eculizumab. Nephrol Dial Transplant 2014;29(3):565–72.
72. Lynn RM, O'Brien SJ, Taylor CM, et al. Childhood hemolytic uremic syndrome, United Kingdom and Ireland. Emerg Infect Dis 2005;11(4):590–6.

73. Garg AX, Suri RS, Barrowman N, et al. Long-term renal prognosis of diarrhea-associated hemolytic uremic syndrome: a systematic review, meta-analysis, and meta-regression. JAMA 2003;290(10):1360–70.
74. Garg AX, Salvadori M, Okell JM, et al. Albuminuria and estimated GFR 5 years after Escherichia coli O157 hemolytic uremic syndrome: an update. Am J Kidney Dis 2008;51(3):435–44.
75. Thajudeen B, Sussman A, Bracamonte E. A case of atypical hemolytic uremic syndrome successfully treated with eculizumab. Case Rep Nephrol Urol 2013; 3(2):139–46.

Thrombotic Microangiopathy

Focus on Atypical Hemolytic Uremic Syndrome

C. John Sperati, MD, MHS[a],*, Alison R. Moliterno, MD[b]

KEYWORDS

- Thrombotic microangiopathy • Atypical hemolytic uremic syndrome
- Hemolytic uremic syndrome • Thrombotic thrombocytopenic purpura

KEY POINTS

- Thrombotic microangiopathies (TMA) are a diverse group of diseases with distinct as well as overlapping pathophysiologic mechanisms.
- TMA is a multifactorial disease, and depends on the relative strengths of constitutional predisposition and external triggers.
- Atypical hemolytic uremic syndrome is characterized by dysregulated activity of the alternative pathway of complement for which blockade at C5 is an effective therapy.
- Owing to heterogeneity in pathophysiology, therapy for TMA must be individualized. An individual patient may exhibit multiple mechanisms of disease.

CASE PRESENTATION

A 31-year-old female presented at 20.2 weeks gestation with fever, dyspnea, acute kidney injury (creatinine, 1.9 mg/dL), dusky painful fingertips, red cell fragmentation, and a platelet count of 7000 cells/mm³. On the second hospital day, she delivered a nonviable fetus. Continuous venovenous hemodialysis was initiated, and laboratory studies were notable for mildly prolonged coagulation times, hypofibrinogenemia, and D-dimer greater than 30 mg/L. A disintegrin and metalloproteinase with a thrombospondin type 1 motif, member 13 (ADAMTS13) activity was 41% (normal, 70%–155%) and complement C3 and C4 were normal. Despite improving with supportive care, she developed seizures on hospital day 10. The C3 was now low at 70 mg/dL (normal, 79–152), and therapeutic plasma exchange (TPE) was initiated. Over the next

Disclosures: The authors have nothing to disclose.
[a] Division of Nephrology, Department of Medicine, The Johns Hopkins University School of Medicine, 1830 East Monument Street, Room 416, Baltimore, MD 21205, USA; [b] Division of Hematology, Department of Medicine, The Johns Hopkins University School of Medicine, 720 Rutland Avenue, Ross 1025, Baltimore, MD 21205, USA
* Corresponding author.
E-mail address: jsperati@jhmi.edu

2 weeks, she received daily TPE with recovery of both platelets and renal function, and ADAMTS13 activity normalized. After discontinuation of TPE, however, platelets and renal function worsened, and ADAMTS13 activity fell to 19%. TPE was reinitiated, and rituximab was administered. Renal biopsy obtained 48 days after her presentation revealed focal cortical infarction, congested glomeruli with loss of capillary endothelial cells, mesangiolysis with embedded erythrocyte fragments, and intimal edema with endothelial activation in an interlobular artery. Immunofluorescence was notable for segmental granular mesangial immunoglobulin (Ig)A (sparse 1–2+), IgM (1+), C3 (1+), kappa (1–2+), and lambda (sparse trace – 1+). Segmental capillary wall staining for C3 (1–3+) was present, and electron microscopy revealed subendothelial widening, capillary loop collapse, and endothelial cell swelling with no electron dense deposits. Platelets and renal function normalized after 29 plasma exchanges. Relevant serologic testing for antinuclear antibodies, antiphospholipid antibody syndrome, and human immunodeficiency virus was negative. Nine months after her presentation, genetic testing identified a heterozygous pathogenic mutation in thrombomodulin (*THBD*; c.1456G>T; p.Asp486Tyr), and a previously unreported heterozygous mutation in complement factor H related protein-5 (*CFHR5*; c.1357C>G; p.Pro453Ala) of unknown significance, consistent with a diagnosis of atypical hemolytic uremic syndrome. Two years later she remains in remission with serum creatinine 0.7 mg/dL (estimated glomerular filtration rate, >60 mL/min/1.73 m^2), normal urine protein excretion, and normal hematologic parameters.

CLASSIFICATION OF THROMBOTIC MICROANGIOPATHY

This case demonstrates the complexity of thrombotic microangiopathy (TMA) syndromes and the challenges clinicians face in arriving at a diagnosis and delivering targeted therapy. TMAs are clinical syndromes defined acutely by the presence of fragmented red cells, anemia, thrombocytopenia (<150,000 cells/mm^3), and microvascular thrombi, with end-organ dysfunction attributed to small vessel occlusion.[1] Chronic, smoldering TMA, particularly renal limited, may not exhibit significant anemia and thrombocytopenia.[2,3] Clinically, TMA is most commonly represented by thrombotic thrombocytopenic purpura (TTP), enteric infection-associated hemolytic uremic syndrome (HUS), complement-mediated atypical HUS (aHUS), and disseminated intravascular coagulation. Many clinical syndromes, however, are characterized by 1 or more of these features, including this patient in whom disseminated intravascular coagulation secondary to fetal demise was initially considered.

Moschcowitz' 1924 report of a 16-year-old with TTP was followed decades later by Gasser's description of HUS in a group of children following diarrheal illness.[4,5] The link between enteric infection by *Escherichia coli* and HUS was established in the 1980s, and molecular diagnostics have firmly established the role of complement dysregulation in the pathogenesis of aHUS.[6–9] Classification rubrics, however, are challenging, given the large number of conditions associated with TMA, the inconsistent use of terminology, and the recognition of overlapping features in these diseases. Many would agree that TTP is characterized by deficiency of ADAMTS13 (activity classically < 5%–10% in TTP), HUS by the presence of Shiga or Shiga-like toxin producing enteric infection (STEC-HUS), and aHUS by complement-mediated disease with the frequent identification of complement-related mutations. Nonetheless, the list of TMA-associated conditions is long (**Box 1**).

Histologically, TMA may be indistinguishable among the different etiologies, with biopsy findings of endothelial injury and thrombus formation, and in the kidney, both intravascular and intraglomerular fibrin thrombi.[10,11] In the acute phase of aHUS, vessels

---

Box 1
Differential diagnosis of thrombotic microangiopathies

A disintegrin and metalloproteinase with a thrombospondin type 1 motif, member 13 (ADAMTS13) deficiency

Thrombotic thrombocytopenic purpura

Infection associated

Shiga or Shiga-like toxin hemolytic uremic syndrome (HUS, typical HUS, Shiga-toxin–associated HUS)

Campylobacter jejuni

Streptococcus pneumonia

Human immunodeficiency virus

Cytomegalovirus

Epstein–Barr virus

Parvovirus B19

BK virus

Influenza

Abnormality in complement regulation

Atypical hemolytic uremic syndrome

Disseminated intravascular coagulation

Autoimmune/connective tissue disease

Systemic lupus erythematosus

Antiphospholipid antibody syndrome

Scleroderma

Vasculitis/glomerulonephritis

Antineutrophil cytoplasmic antibody-associated vasculitis

Membranous nephropathy

Immunoglobulin A nephropathy

Cryoglobulinemia

Pregnancy

Malignant hypertension

Drugs

$P2Y_{12}$ antagonists

Calcineurin inhibitors/sirolimus/everolimus

Quinine

Estrogen/progesterone

Gemcitabine/mitomycin C

Interferon

Vascular endothelial growth factor inhibitors/tyrosine kinase inhibitors

Cocaine

OPANA[R]ER

Metabolic/cell signaling

  Cobalamin responsive methylmalonic acidemia

  Diacylglycerolkinase epsilon mutation

Malignancy

Post organ transplant

display intravascular fibrin thrombi and endothelial swelling and activation, leading to vascular obstruction. Chronically, the glomerular changes may evolve into a membranoproliferative-appearing pattern, although immunofluorescence is often negative for immunoglobulins and electron dense deposits are absent. Chronic vascular changes include vessel wall sclerosis and organizing thrombi, with subendothelial widening and deposition of flocculent material. In contrast, however, to aHUS histology, TTP is characterized by microvascular thrombi rich in platelets, fibrin, and von Willebrand factor (vWF) protein. TTP histology may not invoke the same degree of endothelial damage and edema as aHUS, although the histologic appearance of these 2 diseases often overlaps. The renal microvasculature is relatively spared in TTP, and although acute kidney injury is common in TTP, the creatinine is often less than 2.2 mg/dL and the need for renal replacement therapy occurs in less than 30% of patients.[12–15] Despite the decline in ADAMTS13 activity in our patient, the activity greater than 10% and severity of TMA histology evident on biopsy were most supportive of aHUS.

EPIDEMIOLOGY

Diagnostic uncertainty has confounded epidemiologic, natural history, molecular, and therapeutic studies to this day. The true incidence of TMA is unknown, although 2005 data from the Oklahoma TTP-HUS Registry provide a standardized estimate of suspected TTP-HUS of 11.29 per million per year, with a standardized incidence rate of 1.78 from the most recent 2013 data for confirmed ADAMTS13 deficient TTP.[16,17] Non–diarrheal-associated HUS (presumably aHUS) in children has been estimated at 2 per million.[18] Clinical experience suggests that the diagnosis of TMA, and aHUS in particular, has often been missed. Patients with TMA syndromes typically present during an acute phase requiring hospitalization, and thus hospital-based registries are reasonable sources to capture new cases. **Fig. 1** shows the distribution

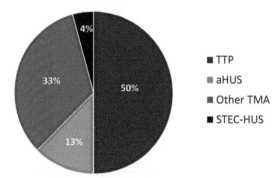

Fig. 1. Distribution of thrombotic microangiopathies (TMA) syndromes in patients recruited in 2014 to the Johns Hopkins Thrombotic Microangiopathies Registry. aHUS, atypical hemolytic uremic syndrome; STEC-HUS, Shiga-toxin–associated hemolytic uremic syndrome; TTP, thrombotic thrombocytopenic purpura.

of TMA from the last 24 adult inpatients recruited in 2014 to the Johns Hopkins TMA Registry. The case under discussion is not included in these data. In this series, classical TTP (defined by a low ADATMS13 [<15%] at initial presentation) comprised more than one-half of TMA, whereas STEC-HUS or typical HUS comprised the minority. Owing to logistical reasons, posttransplant TMA was underrecruited. In our series, one-half of the TTP cases were relapsed episodes; therefore, non-TTP TMA outnumbered new TTP 2 times to 1, a statistic that should inform clinicians considering TMA diagnostics. Originally considered a disease of childhood, 40% to 60% of aHUS actually presents after the age of 18, with only 50% of carriers developing disease by age 45.[19–21] Female predominance is present in TTP and aHUS, representing more than 50% to 75% of cases (**Table 1**).[19,21,22] Infection is a common trigger for aHUS, and in women, pregnancy associates with disease in 20% (**Table 2**).[23] TTP most commonly presents in the second and third trimesters, in part facilitated by the physiologic decline in ADAMTS13 activity with gestation.[24] With aHUS, however, 79% occurred in the postpartum period in the largest series to date.[23] The clinical phenotypes of TTP and aHUS are otherwise frequent mimics, and it is well-recognized that neurologic symptoms are as common in both. Female predominance in both TTP and non-TTP TMA has not been explained adequately, although many of the triggers associated with TMA—autoimmunity, collagen/vascular disorders, and pregnancy—are gender specific. A high prevalence of hypertension and diabetes is noted in all TMA (see **Table 2**), and in this series hypertension preceded the diagnosis of TMA in the majority of cases. Comorbidities may drive TMA or act as risk factors for the development of TMA, and in many patients, it is unclear as to the degree of their causal relationship (see **Table 2**). In the 11 non-TTP, non–STEC-HUS patients evaluated, only 3 were considered to be truly sporadic, whereas 8 were associated with diseases or clinical contexts in which TMA commonly occurs; hence, the classification of "aHUS" (3 patients) and "Other TMA" (8 patients) adopted in the Tables and Figures. TMA is a multifactorial disease, and depends on the relative strengths of constitutional predisposition and external triggers. Strong triggers, such as toxin-associated colitis, may drive HUS in individuals with minimal or no genetic risks, whereas weaker triggers, such as calcineurin inhibitor exposure, may drive disease in those with strong predisposing risks.[25]

In our case, the adult age at presentation would historically have argued against a constitutional disorder of complement regulation, a feature now recognized to be incorrect. Moreover, the reduced ADAMTS13 level during her disease relapse is consistent, in our center's experience, with the spectrum of disease attributable at

Table 1
Demographic features of patients recruited in 2014 to the Johns Hopkins Thrombotic Microangiopathy Registry

	N	Age (Range)	Female	Black Race	Relapse
TTP	12	39 (26–64)	5/12	11/12	6/12
aHUS	3	53 (46–62)	2/3	0/3	0/3
Other TMA	8	48 (24–69)	6/8	5/8	0/8
STEC-HUS	1	84	1/1	0/1	0/1
Total	24	46 (24–84)	14/24	16/24	6/24

Abbreviations: aHUS, atypical hemolytic uremic syndrome; Other TMA, TMA other than TTP, aHUS, STEC-HUS, or disseminated intravascular coagulation; TTP, thrombotic thrombocytopenic purpura; STEC-HUS, Shiga-toxin associated hemolytic uremic syndrome.

Table 2
Comorbidities in patients recruited in 2014 to the Johns Hopkins Thrombotic Microangiopathy Registry

	HTN/ DM	Collagen Vascular	Cancer	Transplant	Drug	HIV	Pregnancy	Diarrhea
TTP	6/12	0	0	0	0	0	0	0
aHUS	3/3	0	0	0	0	0	0	1/3
Other TMA	4/8	2/8	2/8	2/8 renal, BMT	2/8 quinine, tacrolimus	1/8	1/8	0/11
STEC-HUS	1/1	1/1	0	0	0	0	0	1/1
Total	14/24	3/24	2/24	2/24	2/24	1/24	1/24	2/24

Abbreviations: aHUS, atypical hemolytic uremic syndrome; BMT, bone marrow transplant; HIV, human immunodeficiency virus; HTN/DM, hypertension/diabetes mellitus; STEC-HUS, Shiga-toxin–associated hemolytic uremic syndrome; TMA, thrombotic microangiopathies; TTP, thrombotic thrombocytopenic purpura.

least in part to ADAMTS13 pathology (**Fig. 2**). Because her genetic diagnosis is recognized to be in the causal pathway for aHUS (vide infra), her illness can be recast as a strong predisposition to developing aHUS, ultimately triggered by the additional risk factor of pregnancy.

COMPLEMENT PATHWAY AND REGULATION

Complement is a cascading network of proteins critical to innate immunity in defense against microorganisms, clearance of immune complexes, mediation of inflammation, and in embryonic and fetal development.[26–28] Complement is regulated elegantly at multiple levels to minimize excessive activation and bystander injury. The early

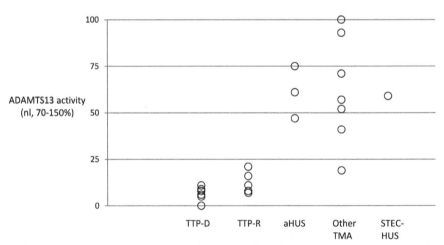

Fig. 2. A disintegrin and metalloproteinase with a thrombospondin type 1 motif, member 13 (ADAMTS13) activity in patients recruited in 2014 to the Johns Hopkins Thrombotic Microangiopathy Registry. aHUS, atypical hemolytic uremic syndrome; STEC-HUS, Shiga-toxin–associated hemolytic uremic syndrome; TMA, thrombotic microangiopathies; TTP, thrombotic thrombocytopenic purpura; TTP-D, patients with first episode of TTP; TTP-R, prevalent TTP patients with relapsed disease.

complement cascade is traditionally initiated via the classical, mannose-binding lectin, or alternative pathway, culminating in the formation of the C5 convertase with subsequent generation of the terminal complement complex C5b-9. C5b-9 forms a membrane-spanning pore capable of inducing sublethal and lethal cellular injury when regulatory control is absent. The prototypical example of C5b-9–mediated lethality of autologous cells is paroxysmal nocturnal hemoglobinuria, characterized by absent cell surface expression of complement regulators CD55 and CD59 owing to loss of their tethering glycophosphatidylinositol anchor. Nontraditional mechanisms for complement activation are now recognized, including thrombin-mediated cleavage of C5 to generate C5b-9 independent of early complement activation.[29] Although all pathways of complement activation have the potential to injure tissue via generation of inflammatory anaphylatoxins C3a and C5a in addition to C5b-9, it is dysregulation of the alternative pathway that has received the greatest attention in the development of aHUS. Classical and mannose-binding lectin–based pathways were believed to likely be of particular relevance to other TMAs, such as seen in systemic lupus erythematosus, antiphospholipid antibody syndrome, and antibody-mediated allograft rejection. Nonetheless, recent data suggest that approximately 82% of kidney biopsies from a small series of aHUS patients contain immunohistochemical evidence of classical and/or mannose-binding lectin activation.[30] These mechanisms of TMA and their particular relevance to aHUS, however, remain inadequately studied.

Initiation of the alternative pathway begins with hydrolysis—either spontaneous or triggered by contact with biological surfaces—of soluble phase C3 to C3(H_2O).[31–33] Hydrolyzed C3 can bind to factor B (CFB), which in the presence of factor D, is cleaved to C3(H_2O)Bb. This soluble phase C3 convertase is stabilized and amplified by properdin, accelerating cleavage of additional C3 to C3b and the anaphylatoxin C3a. The C3 convertase is under negative regulation by factors H (CFH) and I (CFI). Binding of CFH to C3b prevents CFB binding, and also serves as a substrate for CFI-mediated cleavage and inactivation of C3b to iC3b. C3(H_2O) has a slightly higher affinity for CFB than for CFH, favoring formation over degradation of the soluble C3 convertase.[34] There exists a superfamily of Complement Factor H Related Proteins (CFHR1-5) located downstream of CFH in the Regulation of Complement Activation gene cluster on chromosome 1q32. The specific roles of CFHR proteins in complement regulation are loosely understood, but in part may serve as competitive inhibitors of CFH binding.[35] Homozygous deletion of the gene region encompassing *CFHR3* and *CFHR1* is associated with the development of autoantibodies to CFH and the development of aHUS.[36,37] The loss of *CFHR1* may be the critical gene region. Activated C3b covalently links to the cell surface, where it can form surface-bound C3 convertase (C3bBb). Additional C3b binding to the C3 convertase forms the surface bound C5 convertase C3bBbC3b, which is capable of cleaving C5 to soluble C5a and surface-bound C5b. This leads to formation of the pore-forming membrane attack complex (MAC; C5b-9) via assembly of C5b with C6–C9. Some fraction of MAC may be liberated into the soluble phase (sMAC).

Additional surface phase regulation of the complement cascade is provided by cell surface-expressed complement receptor 1 (CR1), decay accelerating factor (DAF; CD55), membrane cofactor protein (MCP; CD46), thrombomodulin (THBD), and CD59. CR1 binds C3b and C4b (classical pathway), thereby facilitating clearance of opsonized particles as well as abrogating activity of the C3/C5 convertases. Both DAF and MCP facilitate C3/C5 convertase disassembly. THBD—mutated in the case under discussion—is an endothelial surface protein that facilitates thrombin activation of activated protein C, inhibits thrombin cleavage of C5, promotes activation of thrombin-activatable fibrinolysis inhibitor (TAFI; carboxypeptidase B) to inactivate

C3a and C5a, and facilitates CFI-mediated inhibition of C3b.[38–40] CD59 antagonizes C9 insertion into C5b-8. In conjunction with soluble vitronectin and clusterin, which also impair C5b-9 assembly, a final opportunity for cell protection against MAC-induced cytotoxicity is provided. Notably, some coagulation factors may function to downregulate complement as well, with plasminogen (PLG) binding C3, C3b, and C5. PLG enhances CFI activity, and activated plasmin is capable of cleaving C5 and C3b at sites distinct from CFI.[41]

MAINTENANCE OF ENDOTHELIAL HEALTH

It is recognized increasingly that the maintenance of endothelial health, as highlighted by the case under discussion, lays at the intersection of complement, coagulation, cell-mediated immunity, and state of endothelial activation. TMA does not develop in the context of a single stimulus (see **Box 1**, **Tables 1** and **2**). Endothelial injury and activation occur through a variety of mechanisms, including trauma, ischemia–reperfusion injury, drug-induced toxicity, infection, shear stress, free heme, complement activation, and inborn errors of cellular metabolism and signaling. Rather than progressing in an orderly, linear fashion, the pathogenesis of TMA incorporates multiple intersecting, simultaneous, and ultimately amplifying pathways.

The predilection of TMA, and particularly complement-mediated injury, for the kidney remains unanswered. The renal microcirculation is distinct from most other vascular beds by virtue of a unique glycocalyx structure and fenestrated endothelium.[42] Glomerular endothelial cells are critically dependent on vascular endothelial growth factor secreted by podocytes, with loss of such signaling (eg, administration of vascular endothelial growth factor antagonists, injury to the glomerular filtration barrier) associated with development of TMA. Moreover, podocytes are a source for complement components, potentially providing another mechanism for amplification of complement-mediated injury during activated states.[43] Endothelial activation upregulates surface expression of vWF, tissue factor, and adhesion molecules such as P-selectin and intercellular adhesion molecule. Complement activation on the surface of platelets and activated endothelium generates the potent anaphylatoxins C3a and C5a, resulting in neutrophil recruitment and activation. Activated neutrophils adhere to the endothelium and migrate into tissue, resulting in further injury as well as disruption of basement membrane integrity through secretion of mediators such as tumor necrosis factor-α.[44] Complement-stimulated neutrophils also increase production of prothrombotic tissue factor.[45,46] THBD transcription and expression is downregulated in endothelial cells under many of these same stimuli, favoring complement activation and coagulation.[40] These changes to the endothelium promote platelet adhesion and generation of microthrombi. The resultant hemolysis and liberation of heme directly activates C3 in the soluble phase, in addition to decreasing expression of surface phase regulators CD46 and CD55.[47] In a potentially protective manner, activated platelets release CFH.[48,49] Impaired CFH activity, however, as a consequence of mutation or inhibitory autoantibody, may activate platelets. Moreover, the endothelial expression of vWF from intracellular Weibel–Palade bodies is accompanied by secretion of co-localized CFH.[50,51] Although increased vWF expression increases platelet adhesion, vWF-bound CFH can augment CFI-mediated complement inhibition. This complement-regulating pathway is lost with deficient CFH activity, thereby increasing both platelet adhesion and complement activation. Endothelial injury may also associate with decreased ADAMTS13 activity, because a large fraction of the ADAMTS13 enzyme is bound to endothelium, reinforcing the connection between endothelial injury, coagulation, and platelet activation (see **Fig. 2**; **Table 3**).

Table 3
Diagnostic and therapeutic features in patients recruited in 2014 to the Johns Hopkins Thrombotic Microangiopathy Registry

Diagnosis	N	Mean ADAMTS13 Activity % (Range)	RRT	TPE	Eculizumab	Presence of Complement Mutations[a]
TTP[b]	6	5.5 (0–11)	0/6	6/6	0/6	0/2
aHUS	3	61 (47–75)	1/3	3/3	3/3	2/3
Other TMA	8	67 (19–100)	4/8	5/8	5/8	4/4
STEC-HUS	1	59	1/1	1/1	1/1	0/1

Abbreviations: aHUS, atypical hemolytic uremic syndrome; ADAMTS13, a disintegrin and metalloproteinase with a thrombospondin type 1 motif, member 13; RRT, renal replacement therapy required; STEC-HUS, Shiga-toxin–associated hemolytic uremic syndrome; TMA, thrombotic microangiopathies; TPE, therapeutic plasma exchange; TTP, thrombotic thrombocytopenic purpura.
[a] Variants identified in the 2014 Thrombotic Microangiopathy Registry are highlighted in bold in **Table 4**.
[b] Relapsed TTP patients excluded from this analysis.

COMPLEMENT DYSREGULATION ASSOCIATED WITH ATYPICAL HEMOLYTIC UREMIC SYNDROME

Although the precise etiology of HUS in general was unknown for many years, the research pendulum swung heavily toward complement-dependent mechanisms of disease in the past 10 years. Demonstration of mutations in complement regulatory genes in aHUS patients has validated this disease paradigm (see **Table 3**; **Table 4**). Moreover, the only therapy approved by the US Food and Drug Administration for

Table 4
Major gene and autoantibody association with atypical hemolytic uremic syndrome

Variant[a]	Frequency (%)
CFH	20–30
CFI	4–10
CD46	5–15
C3	2–10
CFB	1–4
THBD	3–5
CFHR5	<5
CFHR3-CFHR1 deletion	5–15
CFHR1-CFHR4 deletion	N/A
CFH-CFHR1 fusion	3–5
CFH-CFHR3 fusion	N/A
PLG	N/A
DGKE	N/A
ADAMTS13	N/A
Factor H autoantibody	6–10

Abbreviation: ADAMTS13, a disintegrin and metalloproteinase with a thrombospondin type 1 motif, member 13.
[a] Bold indicates variants identified in the presented case and 2014 Thrombotic Microangiopathies Registry case series.
Data from Refs.[19,20,54–61]

aHUS is the C5 antagonist eculizumab, which reduces C5 cleavage and attenuates the terminal complement pathway.[52,53] Not surprisingly, most mutations traditionally associated with aHUS involve inactivation of complement regulatory proteins (see **Table 4**). Notable exceptions are activating mutations in *C3* and *CFB*. *CFH* mutations are most common, but still only represent 30% or less of aHUS. Most *CFH* mutations result in reduced activity with normal plasma concentration, with mutations in short consensus repeats 19 and 20 of the C-terminus being particularly significant.[54] Importantly, mutations in these repeats impair CFH binding to the cell surface, thereby limiting surface phase regulation of complement while leaving soluble phase regulation intact. C3 concentration may be normal in 50% to 70% of patients with aHUS, often reflecting this preserved soluble phase regulation of complement activation. In distinction to this are the activating mutations in *C3* and *CFB*, which result in ongoing soluble phase activation and reduced C3 concentration in 70% to 100% of affected individuals.[9] Additional associated etiologies include autoantibodies directed against CFH, novel CFH–CFHR1 and CFH-CFHR3 fusion proteins, copy number variation of the *CFHR3-CFHR1* and *CFHR1-CFHR4* loci, mutations in clusterin, and potentially autoantibody to CFI, although this remains unconfirmed.[19,20,54–61] In the case under discussion, the patient was heterozygous for the pathogenic c.1456G>T; p.Asp486Tyr mutation in *THBD*, located in the extracellular serine-threonine–rich domain.[40,62] The role of the concomitant *CFHR5* mutation is unknown. The precise function of CFHR5 is uncertain, although by competing with CFH for binding sites it may serve to limit downregulation of complement.[35] The reader is referred to several outstanding reviews on the spectrum of complement mutations in aHUS.[9,63,64]

Although complement-dependent mechanisms of disease in aHUS remain valid, the recognition of alternative mechanisms that may not primarily involve complement serve as a reminder to the complexity of maintaining healthy endothelium. Specific examples, among others, include infantile HUS owing to mutations in diacylglycerol-kinase epsilon, cobalamin-responsive methylmalonic acidemia, and pharmacologic inhibition of vascular endothelial growth factor signaling.[58,65–68] In our series, complement genetic lesions were identified in both aHUS and other non-TTP, non–STEC-HUS TMA (see **Tables 3** and **4**). In our patient, who was ultimately diagnosed with 2 genetic variants in complement-related proteins, a precise measure of complement activity was not available, and measurement of complement components C3, although low, and C4 did not greatly inform her diagnosis.

COMPLEMENT–COAGULATION INTERFACE

A growing body of literature supports the role of altered coagulation in some patients with aHUS. Mutations in *THBD* are an identified cause of aHUS, and a recent exome study of genes involved in the complement and coagulation cascades in 36 patients with aHUS identified 70% to possess either disease related variants or predicted deleterious variants.[60,62] Seven of 8 patients possessing coagulation variants also possessed mutations in complement proteins. Interestingly, 4 of 36 of these patients (11%) possessed variants in *PLG* encoding plasminogen, of which 3 variants have been previously linked to PLG deficiency. The role, however, of PLG in TMA has not been defined clearly. One study of aHUS kidney biopsies has demonstrated increased mRNA expression of plasminogen activator inhibitor-1 and THBD with decreased plasminogen activator expression, suggesting a role for altered fibrinolysis in aHUS. This study, however, was unable to of establish temporality.[69] Studies in childhood diarrhea-associated HUS, however, are at odds regarding the role of impaired fibrinolysis.[70–72] Plasmin, as noted, may downregulate complement activation at the level of

C3 and C5. Recent work has also identified plasmin as capable of degrading platelet–vWF complexes, a potentially important protective role in classical TTP given the absence of adequate ADAMTS13 activity in that disease.[73] Although systemically increased circulating levels of vWF multimers are not a hallmark of aHUS, the presence of ultralarge vWF multimers on endothelial cells provides an activating surface for the assembly of C3 convertase.[74] ADAMTS13 activity in aHUS may be sufficient to prevent the development of a classical TTP phenotype, but its frequently reduced activity may be a contributor to disease pathogenesis (see **Fig. 2** and **Table 3**).[60,75–77]

Small series have reported *ADAMTS13* variants in as many as 50% of aHUS patients, although only a small proportion of these have been investigated and deemed functionally significant.[60,77] Reduced ADAMTS13 activity could enable increased platelet adhesion to the endothelium, while simultaneously providing a surface for complement activation. The presence of plasminogen deficiency—either genetically or secondary to the disease process itself—may synergize with reduced ADAMTS13 activity to provide a mechanism for coagulation–complement induction and propagation of microangiopathy.

FUNCTIONAL ANALYSIS OF COMPLEMENT IN MANAGEMENT OF ATYPICAL HEMOLYTIC UREMIC SYNDROME

Applying the analysis of functional complement activity in the evaluation of aHUS remains challenging. C3 concentration is often normal. Measurement of complement activity via commonly utilized assays such as CH50, AH50, and the Wieslab system (Wieslab Complement System; Euro Diagnostica, Malmö, Sweden) may be normal, and C5a and sMAC may be increased in 47% to 100% and 53% to 100% of acute aHUS, respectively.[77–81] Thus, normal C5a and sMAC concentrations may not exclude the diagnosis of aHUS. Although activated complement products are generally present at greater concentration in aHUS compared with TTP, they are often increased in TTP nonetheless.[80] Soluble phase generation of sMAC may persist during therapy with eculizumab, albeit at reduced levels compared with active disease, although surface deposition of C5b-9 seems to be inhibited.[78] There is no currently available clinical assay for the routine measurement of surface deposited C5b-9. Although the standard CH50 can be used to exclude the rare occurrence of C5 polymorphisms that prevent eculizumab binding or to document terminal pathway inhibition in patients requiring higher doses, the CH50 results do not necessarily correlate well with disease activity, whether on or off therapy.[78,82,83] Traditional markers of complement activation frequently remain elevated in aHUS patients in remission, as well as in unaffected gene carriers. As such, there exists a need for routinely available, easy to perform clinical assays to measure the functional significance of complement activation to separate active from remitted disease.

TRANSLATING DISEASE PHENOTYPING TO TARGETED THERAPY: CHALLENGES AND OPPORTUNITIES

Slow turnaround time for ADAMTS13 activity, limited utility of C3 quantitation, variably informative complement activation studies, delays in renal biopsy, inaccessibility of complement genetic testing, and limited insight into consequences of genetic lesions—counterbalanced with rapidly progressive and morbid diseases—make for an uncomfortable situation. Absent a compelling diagnosis at presentation, given these forces, empiric TPE while awaiting ADAMTS13 activity remains a valid approach. Duration of TPE and possible initiation of complement blockade can be guided by ADAMTS13 activity and clinical response (see **Fig. 2** and **Table 3**). The historical outcome of aHUS treated with TPE alone is poor, with 40% to 60% of patients often reaching end-stage renal disease or death by 1 year. The prompt use of eculizumab can be lifesaving.[19,20,53,84] Clinical presentations most consistent with aHUS should be treated initially with eculizumab while the appropriate diagnostic workup is undertaken. A dosing regimen of 900 mg administered intravenously weekly for 4 weeks, followed by 1200 mg in week 5, and then 1200 mg every 2 weeks thereafter is used in most patients. Occasionally, patients with a larger volume of distribution (eg, pregnant women) may require larger and/or more frequent dosing. All patients should receive vaccination against Neiserria meningitidis, and if administered less than 2 weeks before initiation of eculizumab, antibiotic prophylaxis with a penicillin or fluoroquinolone should be given for 2 weeks after vaccination.[52] It is important to recognize that the currently licensed meningococcal vaccine in the United States (Menactra, Sanofi Pasteur Inc, Swiftwater, PA) does not cover serogroup B, and patients receiving eculizumab remain at risk for meningococcal disease despite vaccination. Some prescribers opt to continue antibiotic prophylaxis indefinitely despite vaccination, but the merits of this approach have not been studied. Streptococcus pneumonia and Haemophilus influenza type b vaccinations should be administered in accordance with the Advisory Committee on Immunization Practices guidelines.

The efficacy of eculizumab in treating aHUS has been demonstrated in 2 phase II clinical trials and a growing literature of case reports and series.[53] In trial 1, 17 participants (41% had a renal transplant) with progressive TMA despite ongoing TPE were administered eculizumab for 26 weeks with primary endpoints of change in platelet count and normalization of hematologic values (ie, normalization of platelet count and lactate dehydrogenase for 2 consecutive measurements over 4 weeks). Participants were eligible for a follow-up extension study with ongoing eculizumab administration. The median duration between diagnosis of aHUS and screening for trial enrollment was 9.7 months. A statistically significant increase in platelet count was seen by day 7, with a median increase in platelet count from baseline to week 26 of 73,000 cells/mm^3 (95% CI, 40,000–105000; P<.001). Eighty-two percent of patients had normalization of platelet count and 76% achieved normal hematologic values by week 26, with 88% achieving both normal platelet counts and hematologic values by week 64 of treatment. The mean increase in the estimated glomerular filtration rate was 32 mL/min/1.73 m^2 (95% CI, 14–49; P = .001), with 4 of 5 dialysis-dependent participants at enrollment stopping renal replacement therapy. In trial 2, 20 participants (40% had a renal transplant) with TPE-dependent TMA without decrease in platelet count for at least 8 weeks were administered eculizumab for 26 weeks with subsequent follow-up in the extension arm. The median duration between diagnosis of aHUS and screening was 48.3 months. By week 26, 80% achieved a TMA event-free status as defined by stable platelet count without TPE or new dialysis initiation, and 90% achieved normalization of hematologic values. By week 62, these endpoints were achieved by 85% and 90% of participants, respectively. The mean increase in the estimated glomerular filtration rate was 6 mL/min/1.73 m^2 (95% CI, 3–9; P<.001). In trial 1, 76% of participants had an identifiable complement genetic variant or autoantibody to CFH, as did 70% in trial 2. The response to eculizumab was more robust the shorter the delay between disease onset and drug administration, and the presence or absence of detectable complement variants did not impact outcome. There remains a paucity of published research regarding the effectiveness of eculizumab for each of the identified complement variants. Optimal management of autoantibodies to CFH is undefined, although eculizumab is reported to be effective, as can be TPE with immunosuppression.[85–87] Little is known regarding the efficacy of eculizumab in patients with phenotypes that overlap the coagulation system. Duration of therapy is an additional unresolved aspect in management. Approximately 80% of disease relapses occur in the first year after diagnosis, such that an empirical duration of therapy of at least 6 to 12 months is not unreasonable.[19] With discontinuation of eculizumab, the relapse risk may be particularly high for patients with *CFH* mutations, and many of these individuals may remain on therapy indefinitely.[88] In a study of 10 patients over a cumulative observation period of 95 months, only the 3 individuals with *CFH* mutations experienced relapse. These relapses occurred with 6 weeks of eculizumab discontinuation, were identified promptly through home urine dipstick monitoring for heme, and were treated readily with resumption of eculizumab. These data certainly do not lessen the potential relapse risk of other genetic variants, but do suggest a strategy of close monitoring upon drug discontinuation may be feasible for many patients. The experience in postrenal transplant patients supports the efficacy of eculizumab in both preventing and treating posttransplant recurrence.[89,90]

It is notable that, in both trials, approximately 30% of patients did not achieve the primary endpoints. Clinicians must remain alert to the vagaries of TMA, the unresolved questions in pathogenesis and management, and the recognition that treatment of some etiologies (eg, malignancy, scleroderma renal crisis, malignant hypertension, cobalamin-responsive methylmalonic acidemia) routinely involve neither TPE nor eculizumab at the present time. The presented patient's prolonged course of plasma-based therapy ultimately resulted in complete remission that has been sustained over 2 years later. Although plasma therapy can ameliorate THBD-induced aHUS, 54% of patients were nonetheless deceased or on dialysis by 3 years in 1 series.[20,91,92]

In addition, a reappraisal of adjunct therapies in TMA management is needed. Based on data from childhood HUS, the use of heparin may not be helpful.[93,94] Heparin binding, however, is an important facet of complement regulation, and prevention of microthrombus formation could be advantageous. Data on its use are lacking in aHUS, and although the risk for bleeding must not be minimized, its use may warrant further exploration.[95,96] In addition, the renin–angiotensin–aldosterone pathway is activated owing to renal arteriolar microangiopathy in TMA, and renin–angiotensin–aldosterone antagonism similar to the management approach in scleroderma renal crisis may be appropriate.[97–99] Last, corticosteroids decrease neutrophil activation and decrease complement synthesis, although their effect on the latter is complex and time dependent.[100–102] The role for their use is undefined.

SUMMARY

Atypical HUS is a disease where host risks and triggers interplay, and endothelial damage initiated by the interplay of host and trigger then grows to involve coagulation, fibrinolysis, platelet, and white cell activation. Phenotype modulation by variables such as promoter effects, epigenetics, and other gene products are possible, as nicely illuminated by the case of 2 sisters, both with congenital TTP, in which only 1 carried a concomitant factor H mutation and developed kidney failure.[84,103] As understanding of the diverse mechanisms grows, it has become apparent that a common therapeutic approach to all TMA does not exist. Moreover, therapies beyond TPE and complement inhibitors that address these additional pathways—heparin, renin–angiotensin–aldosterone antagonism, antiplatelet agents, and so on—may have significant roles and need to be revisited. Finally, as further insight is gained into the functional significance of specific variants in complement and coagulation proteins, there is hope that therapies can be tailored for both short-term treatment and long-term prophylaxis. Although the presence of genetic variants does not always imply functional consequence, in this case, the results of genetic testing will help to guide future therapy in the event of relapse.[104,105]

REFERENCES

1. George JN, Nester CM. Syndromes of thrombotic microangiopathy. N Engl J Med 2014;371(7):654–66.
2. Sallée M, Ismail K, Fakhouri F, et al. Thrombocytopenia is not mandatory to diagnose haemolytic and uremic syndrome. BMC Nephrol 2013;14:3.
3. Belingheri M, Possenti I, Tel F, et al. Cryptic activity of atypical hemolytic uremic syndrome and eculizumab treatment. Pediatrics 2014;133(6):e1769–71.
4. Moschcowitz E. Hyaline thrombosis of the terminal arterioles and capillaries: a hitherto undescribed disease. Proc N Y Pathol Soc 1924;24:21–4.
5. Gasser C, Gautier E, Steck A, et al. Hemolytic-uremic syndrome: bilateral necrosis of the renal cortex in acute acquired hemolytic anemia. Schweiz Med Wochenschr 1955;85(38–39):905–9.
6. Cameron JS, Vick R. Letter: plasma-C3 in haemolytic-uraemic syndrome and thrombotic thrombocytopenic purpura. Lancet 1973;2(7835):975.
7. Stühlinger W, Kourilsky O, Kanfer A, et al. Haemolytic-uraemic syndrome: evidence for intravascular C3 activation. Lancet 1974;304(7883):788–9.
8. Warwicker P, Goodship TH, Donne RL, et al. Genetic studies into inherited and sporadic hemolytic uremic syndrome. Kidney Int 1998;53(4):836–44.
9. Loirat C, Frémeaux-Bacchi V. Atypical hemolytic uremic syndrome. Orphanet J Rare Dis 2011;6(1):60.
10. Taylor CM, Chua C, Howie AJ, et al. Clinico-pathological findings in diarrhoea-negative haemolytic uraemic syndrome. Pediatr Nephrol 2004;19(4):419–25.
11. Sethi S, Fervenza FC. Pathology of renal diseases associated with dysfunction of the alternative pathway of complement: C3 glomerulopathy and atypical hemolytic uremic syndrome (aHUS). Semin Thromb Hemost 2014;40(4):416–21.
12. George JN. How I treat patients with thrombotic thrombocytopenic purpura. Blood 2010;116(20):4060–9.
13. Zuber J, Fakhouri F, Roumenina LT, et al. Use of eculizumab for atypical haemolytic uraemic syndrome and C3 glomerulopathies. Nat Rev Nephrol 2012;8(11): 643–57.
14. Coppo P, Schwarzinger M, Buffet M, et al. Predictive features of severe acquired ADAMTS13 deficiency in idiopathic thrombotic microangiopathies: the French TMA reference center experience. PLoS One 2010;5(4):e10208.
15. Zafrani L, Mariotte E, Darmon M, et al. Acute renal failure is prevalent in patients with thrombotic thrombocytopenic purpura associated with low plasma ADAMTS13 activity. J Thromb Haemost 2014. http://dx.doi.org/10.1111/jth. 12826.
16. Terrell DR, Williams LA, Vesely SK, et al. The incidence of thrombotic thrombocytopenic purpura-hemolytic uremic syndrome: all patients, idiopathic patients, and patients with severe ADAMTS-13 deficiency. J Thromb Haemost 2005;3(7): 1432–6.
17. Reese JA, Muthurajah DS, Kremer Hovinga JA, et al. Children and adults with thrombotic thrombocytopenic purpura associated with severe, acquired Adamts13 deficiency: comparison of incidence, demographic and clinical features. Pediatr Blood Cancer 2013;60(10):1676–82.
18. Constantinescu AR, Bitzan M, Weiss LS, et al. Non-enteropathic hemolytic uremic syndrome: causes and short-term course. Am J Kidney Dis 2004;43(6):976–82.

19. Fremeaux-Bacchi V, Fakhouri F, Garnier A, et al. Genetics and outcome of atypical hemolytic uremic syndrome: a nationwide French series comparing children and adults. Clin J Am Soc Nephrol 2013;8(4):554–62.
20. Noris M, Caprioli J, Bresin E, et al. Relative role of genetic complement abnormalities in sporadic and familial aHUS and their impact on clinical phenotype. Clin J Am Soc Nephrol 2010;5(10):1844–59.
21. Sullivan M, Erlic Z, Hoffmann MM, et al. Epidemiological approach to identifying genetic predispositions for atypical hemolytic uremic syndrome. Ann Hum Genet 2010;74(1):17–26.
22. Licht C, Ardissino G, Ariceta G, et al. Characteristics of 406 adult and pediatric patients in the global aHUS registry. American Society of Nephrology Kidney Week, Philadelphia, 2014 [abstract SA-PO510].
23. Fakhouri F, Roumenina L, Provot F, et al. Pregnancy-associated hemolytic uremic syndrome revisited in the era of complement gene mutations. J Am Soc Nephrol 2010;21(5):859–67.
24. Mannucci PM, Canciani MT, Forza I, et al. Changes in health and disease of the metalloprotease that cleaves von Willebrand factor. Blood 2001;98(9):2730–5.
25. Le Quintrec M, Lionet A, Kamar N, et al. Complement mutation-associated de novo thrombotic microangiopathy following kidney transplantation. Am J Transplant 2008;8(8):1694–701.
26. Morgan BP. Complement. In: Paul WE, editor. Fundamental immunology. 7th edition. Philadelphia: Lippincott Williams & Wilkins; 2012.
27. Degn SE, Jensenius JC, Thiel S. Disease-causing mutations in genes of the complement system. Am J Hum Genet 2011;88(6):689–705.
28. Hawksworth OA, Coulthard LG, Taylor SM, et al. Brief report: complement c5a promotes human embryonic stem cell pluripotency in the absence of FGF2. Stem Cells 2014;32(12):3278–84.
29. Huber-Lang M, Sarma JV, Zetoune FS, et al. Generation of C5a in the absence of C3: a new complement activation pathway. Nat Med 2006;12(6):682–7.
30. Chua JS, Baelde HJ, Zandbergen M, et al. Complement Factor C4d Is a Common Denominator in Thrombotic Microangiopathy. J Am Soc Nephrol 2015 [pii:ASN.2014050429].
31. Pangburn MK, Müller-Eberhard HJ. Initiation of the alternative complement pathway due to spontaneous hydrolysis of the thioester of C3. Ann N Y Acad Sci 1983;421:291–8.
32. Nilsson B, Ekdahl KN. The tick-over theory revisited: is C3 a contact-activated protein? Immunobiology 2012;217(11):1106–10.
33. Mathern DR, Heeger PS. Molecules great and small: the complement system. Clin J Am Soc Nephrol 2015 [pii:CJN.06230614].
34. Isenman D, Kells D. Nucleophilic modification of human complement protein C3: correlation of conformational changes with acquisition of C3b-like functional properties. Biochemistry 1981;20(15):4458–67.
35. Skerka C, Chen Q, Fremeaux-Bacchi V, et al. Complement factor H related proteins (CFHRs). Mol Immunol 2013;56(3):170–80.
36. Dragon-Durey MA, Blanc C, Marliot F, et al. The high frequency of complement factor H related CFHR1 gene deletion is restricted to specific subgroups of patients with atypical haemolytic uraemic syndrome. J Med Genet 2009;46(7):447–50.
37. Moore I, Strain L, Pappworth I, et al. Association of factor H autoantibodies with deletions of CFHR1, CFHR3, CFHR4, and with mutations in CFH, CFI, CD46, and C3 in patients with atypical hemolytic uremic syndrome. Blood 2010;115(2):379–87.

38. Nishimura T, Myles T, Piliponsky AM, et al. Thrombin-activatable procarboxy-peptidase B regulates activated complement C5a in vivo. Blood 2007;109(5): 1992–7.

39. Morser J, Gabazza EC, Myles T, et al. What has been learnt from the thrombin-activatable fibrinolysis inhibitor-deficient mouse? J Thromb Haemost 2010;8(5): 868–76.

40. Conway EM. Thrombomodulin and its role in inflammation. Semin Immunopathol 2012;34(1):107–25.

41. Barthel D, Schindler S, Zipfel PF. Plasminogen is a complement inhibitor. J Biol Chem 2012;287(22):18831–42.

42. Boels MG, Lee DH, van den Berg BM, et al. The endothelial glycocalyx as a potential modifier of the hemolytic uremic syndrome. Eur J Intern Med 2013; 24(6):503–9.

43. Sacks SH, Zhou W, Pani A, et al. Complement C3 gene expression and regulation in human glomerular epithelial cells. Immunology 1993;79(3):348–54.

44. Finsterbusch M, Voisin MB, Beyrau M, et al. Neutrophils recruited by chemoattractants in vivo induce microvascular plasma protein leakage through secretion of TNF. J Exp Med 2014;211(7):1307–14.

45. Ritis K, Doumas M, Mastellos D, et al. A novel C5a receptor-tissue factor cross-talk in neutrophils links innate immunity to coagulation pathways. J Immunol 2006;177(7):4794–802.

46. Kambas K, Markiewski MM, Pneumatikos IA, et al. C5a and TNF- up-regulate the expression of tissue factor in intra-alveolar neutrophils of patients with the acute respiratory distress syndrome. J Immunol 2008;180(11):7368–75.

47. Frimat M, Tabarin F, Dimitrov JD, et al. Complement activation by heme as a secondary hit for atypical hemolytic uremic syndrome. Blood 2013;122(2): 282–92.

48. Licht C, Pluthero FG, Li L, et al. Platelet-associated complement factor H in healthy persons and patients with atypical HUS. Blood 2009;114(20):4538–45.

49. Ståhl A, Vaziri-Sani F, Heinen S, et al. Factor H dysfunction in patients with atypical hemolytic uremic syndrome contributes to complement deposition on platelets and their activation. Blood 2008;111(11):5307–15.

50. Rayes J, Roumenina LT, Dimitrov JD, et al. The interaction between factor H and VWF increases factor H cofactor activity and regulates VWF prothrombotic status. Blood 2014;123(1):121–5.

51. Nightingale T, Cutler D. The secretion of von Willebrand factor from endothelial cells; an increasingly complicated story. J Thromb Haemost 2013;11(Suppl 1): 192–201.

52. Soliris [package insert]. Cheshire, CT: Alexion Pharmaceuticals, Inc; 2014.

53. Legendre CM, Licht C, Muus P, et al. Terminal complement inhibitor eculizumab in atypical hemolytic-uremic syndrome. N Engl J Med 2013;368(23):2169–81.

54. Kavanagh D, Goodship TH, Richards A. Atypical hemolytic uremic syndrome. Semin Nephrol 2013;33(6):508–30.

55. Kavanagh D, Pappworth IY, Anderson H, et al. Factor I autoantibodies in patients with atypical hemolytic uremic syndrome: disease-associated or an epiphenomenon? Clin J Am Soc Nephrol 2012;7(3):417–26.

56. Loirat C, Saland J, Bitzan M. Management of hemolytic uremic syndrome. Presse Med 2012;41(3 Pt 2):e115–35.

57. Westra D, Vernon KA, Volokhina EB, et al. Atypical hemolytic uremic syndrome and genetic aberrations in the complement factor H-related 5 gene. J Hum Genet 2012;57(7):459–64.

58. Lemaire M, Frémeaux-Bacchi V, Schaefer F, et al. Recessive mutations in DGKE cause atypical hemolytic-uremic syndrome. Nat Genet 2013;45(5):531–6.
59. Ståhl A, Kristoffersson A, Olin AI, et al. A novel mutation in the complement regulator clusterin in recurrent hemolytic uremic syndrome. Mol Immunol 2009; 46(11–12):2236–43.
60. Bu F, Maga T, Meyer NC, et al. Comprehensive genetic analysis of complement and coagulation genes in atypical hemolytic uremic syndrome. J Am Soc Nephrol 2014;25(1):55–64.
61. Francis NJ, Mcnicholas B, Awan A, et al. A novel hybrid CFH/CFHR3 gene generated by a microhomology-mediated deletion in familial atypical hemolytic uremic syndrome. Blood 2012;119(2):591–601.
62. Delvaeye M, Noris M, De Vriese A, et al. Thrombomodulin mutations in atypical hemolytic-uremic syndrome. N Engl J Med 2009;361(4):345–57.
63. Riedl M, Fakhouri F, Le Quintrec M, et al. Spectrum of complement-mediated thrombotic microangiopathies: pathogenetic insights identifying novel treatment approaches. Semin Thromb Hemost 2014;40(4):444–64.
64. Rodríguez de Córdoba S, Hidalgo MS, Pinto S, et al. Genetics of atypical hemolytic uremic syndrome (aHUS). Semin Thromb Hemost 2014;40(4):422–30.
65. Bruneau S, Néel M, Roumenina LT, et al. Loss of DGKε induces endothelial cell activation and death independently of complement activation. Blood 2015; 125(6):1038–46.
66. Westland R, Bodria M, Carrea A, et al. Phenotypic expansion of DGKE-associated diseases. J Am Soc Nephrol 2014;25(7):1408–14.
67. Cornec-Le Gall E, Delmas Y, De Parscau L, et al. Adult-onset eculizumab-resistant hemolytic uremic syndrome associated with cobalamin C deficiency. Am J Kidney Dis 2014;63(1):119–23.
68. Eremina V, Jefferson JA, Kowalewska J, et al. VEGF inhibition and renal thrombotic microangiopathy. N Engl J Med 2008;358(11):1129–36.
69. Modde F, Agustian PA, Wittig J, et al. Comprehensive analysis of glomerular mRNA expression of pro- and antithrombotic genes in atypical haemolytic-uremic syndrome (aHUS). Virchows Arch 2013;462(4):455–64.
70. Chandler WL, Jelacic S, Boster DR, et al. Prothrombotic coagulation abnormalities preceding the hemolytic-uremic syndrome. N Engl J Med 2002;346(1): 23–32.
71. Van Geet C, Proesmans W, Arnout J, et al. Activation of both coagulation and fibrinolysis in childhood hemolytic uremic syndrome. Kidney Int 1998;54(4): 1324–30.
72. Proesmans W, Geet CV. Fibrinolysis in the hemolytic uremic syndrome. Pediatr Nephrol 2002;17(10):871–2 [author reply: 873–4].
73. Tersteeg C, de Maat S, De Meyer SF, et al. Plasmin cleavage of von Willebrand factor as an emergency bypass for ADAMTS13 deficiency in thrombotic microangiopathy. Circulation 2014;129(12):1320–31.
74. Turner NA, Moake J. Assembly and activation of alternative complement components on endothelial cell-anchored ultra-large von Willebrand factor links complement and hemostasis-thrombosis. PLoS One 2013;8(3):e59372.
75. Furlan M, Robles R, Galbusera M, et al. von Willebrand factor-cleaving protease in thrombotic thrombocytopenic purpura and the hemolytic-uremic syndrome. N Engl J Med 1998;339(22):1578–84.
76. Remuzzi G, Galbusera M, Noris M, et al. von Willebrand factor cleaving protease (ADAMTS13) is deficient in recurrent and familial thrombotic thrombocytopenic purpura and hemolytic uremic syndrome. Blood 2002;100(3):778–85.

77. Feng S, Eyler SJ, Zhang Y, et al. Partial ADAMTS13 deficiency in atypical hemolytic uremic syndrome. Blood 2013;122(8):1487–93.
78. Noris M, Galbusera M, Gastoldi S, et al. Dynamics of complement activation in aHUS and how to monitor eculizumab therapy. Blood 2014;124(11):1715–26.
79. Cugno M, Gualtierotti R, Possenti I, et al. Complement functional tests for monitoring eculizumab treatment in patients with atypical hemolytic uremic syndrome. J Thromb Haemost 2014;12(9):1440–8.
80. Cataland S, Holers V. Biomarkers of terminal complement activation confirm the diagnosis of aHUS and differentiate aHUS from TTP. Blood 2014;123(24):3733–8.
81. Sánchez-Corral P, González-Rubio C, Rodríguez de Córdoba S, et al. Functional analysis in serum from atypical Hemolytic Uremic Syndrome patients reveals impaired protection of host cells associated with mutations in factor H. Mol Immunol 2004;41(1):81–4.
82. Nishimura J, Yamamoto M, Hayashi S, et al. Genetic variants in C5 and poor response to eculizumab. N Engl J Med 2014;370(7):632–9.
83. Jodele S, Fukuda T, Vinks A, et al. Eculizumab therapy in children with severe hematopoietic stem cell transplantation-associated thrombotic microangiopathy. Biol Blood Marrow Transplant 2014;20(4):518–25.
84. Bresin E, Rurali E, Caprioli J, et al. Combined complement gene mutations in atypical hemolytic uremic syndrome influence clinical phenotype. J Am Soc Nephrol 2013;24(3):475–86.
85. Dragon-Durey MA, Sethi SK, Bagga A, et al. Clinical features of anti-factor H autoantibody-associated hemolytic uremic syndrome. J Am Soc Nephrol 2010;21(33):2180–7.
86. Boyer O, Balzamo E, Charbit M, et al. Pulse cyclophosphamide therapy and clinical remission in atypical hemolytic uremic syndrome with anti-complement factor H autoantibodies. Am J Kidney Dis 2010;55(5):923–7.
87. Noone D, Waters A, Pluthero FG, et al. Successful treatment of DEAP-HUS with eculizumab. Pediatr Nephrol 2014;29:841–51.
88. Ardissino G, Testa S, Possenti I, et al. Discontinuation of eculizumab maintenance treatment for atypical hemolytic uremic syndrome: a report of 10 cases. Am J Kidney Dis 2014;64(4):633–7.
89. Zuber J, Le Quintrec M, Krid S, et al. Eculizumab for atypical hemolytic uremic syndrome recurrence in renal transplantation. Am J Transplant 2012;12:3337–54.
90. Matar D, Naqvi F, Racusen LC, et al. Atypical hemolytic uremic syndrome recurrence after kidney transplantation. Transplantation 2014;98(11):1205–12.
91. Honda T, Ogata S, Mineo E, et al. A novel strategy for hemolytic uremic syndrome: successful treatment with thrombomodulin α. Pediatrics 2013;131(3):e928–33.
92. Sánchez Chinchilla D, Pinto S, Hoppe B, et al. Complement mutations in diacylglycerol kinase-ε-associated atypical hemolytic uremic syndrome. Clin J Am Soc Nephrol 2014;9(9):1611–9.
93. Vitacco M, Sanchez Avalos J, Gianantonio CA. Heparin therapy in the hemolytic-uremic syndrome. J Pediatr 1973;83(2):271–5.
94. Loirat C, Beaufils F, Sonsino E, et al. Treatment of childhood hemolytic-uremic syndrome with urokinase. Cooperative controlled trial. Arch Fr Pediatr 1984;41(1):15–9.
95. Michael M, Elliott EJ, Ridley GF, et al. Interventions for haemolytic uraemic syndrome and thrombotic thrombocytopenic purpura. Cochrane Database Syst Rev 2009;(1):CD003595.

96. Girardi G, Redecha P, Salmon JE. Heparin prevents antiphospholipid antibody-induced fetal loss by inhibiting complement activation. Nat Med 2004;10(11): 1222–6.

97. Rocha R, Chander PN, Zuckerman A, et al. Role of aldosterone in renal vascular injury in stroke-prone hypertensive rats. Hypertension 1999;33(1 Pt 2):232–7.

98. Akimoto T, Muto S, Ito C, et al. Clinical features of malignant hypertension with thrombotic microangiopathy. Clin Exp Hypertens 2011;33(2):77–83.

99. Steen VD. Kidney involvement in systemic sclerosis. Presse Med 2014;43(10 Pt 2): e305–14.

100. Atkinson J, Frank M. Effect of cortisone therapy on serum complement components. J Immunol 1973;111(4):1061–6.

101. Hammerschmidt DE, White JG, Craddock PR, et al. Corticosteroids inhibit complement-induced granulocyte aggregation. A possible mechanism for their efficacy in shock states. J Clin Invest 1979;63(4):798–803.

102. Zimmermann-Nielsen E, Grønbaek H, Dahlerup JF, et al. Complement activation capacity in plasma before and during high-dose prednisolone treatment and tapering in exacerbations of Crohn's disease and ulcerative colitis. BMC Gastroenterol 2005;5:31.

103. Noris M, Bucchioni S, Galbusera M, et al. Complement factor H mutation in familial thrombotic thrombocytopenic purpura with ADAMTS13 deficiency and renal involvement. J Am Soc Nephrol 2005;16(5):1177–83.

104. Tortajada A, Pinto S, Martínez-Ara J, et al. Complement factor H variants I890 and L1007 while commonly associated with atypical hemolytic uremic syndrome are polymorphisms with no functional significance. Kidney Int 2012;81(1):56–63.

105. Marinozzi MC, Vergoz L, Rybkine T, et al. Complement factor B mutations in atypical hemolytic uremic syndrome-disease-relevant or benign? J Am Soc Nephrol 2014;25(9):2053–65.

Current and Future Pharmacologic Complement Inhibitors

Antonio M. Risitano, MD, PhD

KEYWORDS

- Eculizumab • Complement therapeutics • PNH • aHUS • C3 • C5 • Compstatin

KEY POINTS

- Eculizumab is the current anticomplement treatment agent approved for the treatment of paroxysmal nocturnal hemoglobinuria and atypical hemolytic uremic syndrome.
- Emerging observations are suggesting that other strategies of complement inhibition/modulation may improve the clinical result of current anticomplement treatment.
- Novel complement therapeutics include inhibitors of the terminal effector complement as well as of early complement activation.
- Inhibitors of early complement inhibitors include broad C3 inhibitors as well as agents selectively targeting specific complement pathways.

INTRODUCTION

The complement system is a key component of innate immunity, which is involved in several physiologic and pathologic processes. It was originally thought that complement merely represents the crudest sentinel for protection from microbes, with a possible additional role in inflammatory processes; however, its role in human homeostasis and disease is now widely recognized.[1–3] Indeed, dysregulated or impaired complement is involved in an increasing list of human diseases (eg, paroxysmal nocturnal hemoglobinuria [PNH], hemolytic uremic syndrome [HUS], kidney disorders, age-related macular degeneration [AMD]) as well as of clinical conditions (eg, sepsis, ischemia/reperfusion injury, allograft rejection).[4] The interest for complement-mediated pathophysiology has been strengthened by the recent availability of

The author has received research funding from Alexion Pharmaceuticals, Amyndas Pharmaceuticals, Alnylam Pharmaceuticals, Rapharma, and Novartis. He is also consultant for Alnylam Pharmaceuticals and Rapharma and a member of an Advisory Board for Alexion.
Bone Marrow Transplantation Clinical Unit, Hematology, Department of Clinical Medicine and Surgery, Federico II University of Naples, Via Pansini 5, Naples 80131, Italy
E-mail address: amrisita@unina.it

Hematol Oncol Clin N Am 29 (2015) 561–582
http://dx.doi.org/10.1016/j.hoc.2015.01.009

complement inhibitors.[5,6] Indeed, the clinical approval of the first complement-targeting drug, the anti-complement component 5 (C5) Eculizumab (Soliris), has drastically changed the natural history PNH and represents a novel treatment option for other complement-mediated diseases, such as atypical hemolytic uremic syndrome (aHUS). Subsequently, the introduction of the C1 inhibitor (C1-INH; Cinryze) for the treatment of hereditary angioedema has offered another compound in the armamentarium for the interception of specific component of the complement cascade.[7] All these observations have reignited the interest for a deeper investigation of complement-mediated pathophysiology in human diseases as well as the interest for the development of novel classes of complement inhibitors. Here, current and future agents are reviewed that intercept complement function in vivo and the rationale for targeted complement inhibition for optimizing the therapeutic effect in specific clinical conditions is discussed.

CURRENT COMPLEMENT INHIBITORS: ECULIZUMAB
Eculizumab for the Treatment of Paroxysmal Nocturnal Hemoglobinuria

PNH is a rare hematologic disease characterized by complement-mediated intravascular hemolysis, bone marrow failure, and propensity to thromboembolic events.[8–10] PNH is due to a somatic mutation in the phosphatidyl-inositol glycan class A (*PIG-A*) gene,[11,12] which impairs the biosynthesis of the glycosyl-phosphatidyl-inositol (GPI) anchor and the subsequent expression of a several surface proteins (GPI-linked proteins). The absence of 2 GPI-anchored complement regulatory proteins (CD55 and C59) is central to the pathophysiology of PNH. CD55 is a regulator of early complement activation,[13] which physiologically inhibits the formation of C3 convertase (both C3bBb and C4b2a) and also promotes its decay.[14] CD59 is a regulator of the terminal effector complement,[15] which interacts with C8 and C9, inhibiting the incorporation of this latter onto the C5b–C8 complex, eventually preventing the assembly of the membrane attack complex (MAC).[16] The concomitant lack of CD55 and CD59 accounts for the susceptibility of PNH erythrocytes to complement activation, which eventually leads to the chronic intravascular hemolysis typical of PNH.

Eculizumab (Soliris) is the first complement inhibitor available in the clinic; it is a humanized monoclonal antibody (mAb),[17] which binds the complement component 5 (C5) and inhibits its cleavage to C5a and C5b, eventually disabling the terminal effector complement (preventing the assembly of the MAC). Eculizumab has been extensively tested in different autoimmune disorders before changing the treatment paradigm of PNH; indeed, 2 large multinational phase III studies demonstrated the efficacy of eculizumab for the treatment of PNH.[18,19] In the first double-blind, placebo-controlled, multinational randomized trial (TRIUMPH), which enrolled 86 transfusion-dependent PNH patients, treatment with eculizumab resulted in a dramatic reduction of intravascular hemolysis, as measured by *lactate dehydrogenase* (LDH), leading to hemoglobin stabilization and transfusion independence in about half of the patients (and reduced transfusional need in the remaining ones).[18] These data were confirmed in the open-label phase III study, SHEPHERD, which included a broader PNH population[19]; this longer study also confirmed the excellent safety profile of eculizumab, with negligible side effects. A subsequent open-label extension study confirmed the efficacy and the safety of eculizumab with a longer follow-up, demonstrating a sustained control of intravascular hemolysis with all related signs and symptoms.[20] This study also demonstrated a remarkable (85%) reduction in the rate of thromboembolic complications,[20] possibly because of the pathogenic linkage between intravascular hemolysis and thrombosis (eg, nitric oxide consumption,[21] prothrombotic microvesicles) or to any direct effect on complement-mediated thrombophilia (ie, on PNH platelets).[22,23] Preliminary data on survival seem to suggest that eculizumab may also improve survival in PNH,[24] as expected given its effect on the main cause of death in PNH (ie, thrombosis). Based on these data, eculizumab is the standard treatment for PNH, already approved in most countries; according to country-specific guidelines, the indication for treatment includes red blood cell transfusion dependency, and possibly, severe recurrent hemolytic paroxysms and life-threatening thrombotic complications.

Hematologic response to eculizumab in paroxysmal nocturnal hemoglobinuria
Irrespective of a remarkable effect on complement-mediated intravascular hemolysis, the hematologic benefit of PNH patients on eculizumab is extremely heterogeneous: indeed, a significant proportion of patients continue to require some blood transfusions.[18,19,25,26] Different factors may be responsible for this insufficient hematologic response to eculizumab.

1. Bone marrow failure is the most obvious reason; it is clearly identified by low/inadequate reticulocyte counts in patients who do not show any laboratory sign of hemolysis, and it may require additional specific treatments (ie, bone marrow transplantation or immunosuppression).[27]
2. A second possible reason is residual intravascular hemolysis; it may appear as "pharmacokinetic breakthrough," recurrently appearing in the few hours preceding the next dosing of eculizumab (10%–15% of patients,[28] who may benefit from changes in dosages of administration interval of eculizumab), or as "pharmacodynamic breakthrough," occurring in concomitance with boosted complement activation (typically at time of infections).
3. A third possible reason is the presence of an intrinsic resistance to eculizumab due to mutated C5; this possibility has been recently demonstrated in a Japanese cohort,[29] but it seems to be restricted to a limited number of patients (and possibly to specific ethnicities).
4. The forth and most common cause of residual anemia during eculizumab treatment is C3-mediated extravascular hemolysis[25]; it is mechanistically related to the pharmacologic effect of eculizumab and pertains to all PNH patients on eculizumab, even if it becomes clinically relevant in about one-third.

C3-mediated extravascular hemolysis Inhibition by eculizumab intercepts the complement cascade at the level of C5, eventually counteracting the lack of CD59 on PNH erythrocytes. However, eculizumab does not affect earlier events in complement activation, and especially those that remain uncontrolled because of the lack of CD55. Thus, PNH erythrocytes, which are spared from MAC-mediated hemolysis, progressively accumulate on their surface C3 fragments, which eventually work as opsonins leading to phagocytosis by liver and spleen macrophages. This mechanism of extravascular hemolysis occurs through the recognition of C3 opsonins by specific complement receptors expressed on phagocytic cells, resulting in a selective destruction of PNH erythrocytes, which have been exposed to threshold complement activation. C3-mediated extravascular hemolysis remains subclinical in most PNH patients on eculizumab, but it results in severe anemia in about one-third of them[25,26,30–32]; recently, it has been reported that a hypofunctional polymorphic variant of complement receptor 1 (CR1) is associated with higher C3 opsonization and lower chance of optimal response to eculizumab.[33] All these findings support a view whereby complement may remain harmful to PNH erythrocytes even during eculizumab treatment, paving the way for the development of novel complement therapeutics.

Eculizumab in Other Indications: Atypical Hemolytic Uremic Syndrome and Cold Agglutinin Disease

Hemolytic uremic syndrome

After its introduction in the clinic, eculizumab was tested in other indications; for the purpose of this review, discussion is limited to hemolytic anemias. Indeed, eculizumab has also been approved for the treatment of HUS, another rare disease that is characterized by thrombotic microangiopathy (TMA), leading to mechanic intravascular hemolytic anemia, platelet consumption, and end-stage renal disease.[34,35] HUS can be distinct in a sporadic (typical) HUS form, which is acquired and usually associated with infectious events (typically by Shiga-toxin-producing *Escherichia coli*, STEC), and an atypical form (aHUS), which is inherited. Indeed, aHUS is associated with inherited mutations of different complement genes, including complement factor H (CFH), complement factor I (CFI), complement factor B (CFB), membrane cofactor protein, thrombomodulin, C3 convertase, and C3,[36–39] clearly pointing out the pathogenic role of complement in this condition.[35] The efficacy of eculizumab in aHUS has been initially demonstrated in 2 distinct prospective trials enrolling aHUS patients who were either resistant to plasma exchange (PE) and/or plasma infusion (PI), or who required PE/PI.[40] In the first trial, which enrolled patients with evidence of platelet consumption, the increase in platelet count was used as efficacy endpoint, as an indicator of ceased TMA. After the initial 26 weeks of treatment, all 17 patients showed some increase in platelet count, with normalization of hematologic values in 88% of patients (15 of 15 who continued to receive the treatment, median treatment duration, 64 weeks). TMA-free status was achieved in 88% of patients (15/17), and only 2 patients required further PE (1 after eculizumab discontinuation due to study withdrawal). More than half of the patients also exhibited a substantial improvement in renal function (as measured by creatinine and GFR), with 4 of 5 patients on dialysis who did not require further procedures.[40] In the second trial, which included 20 aHUS patients on chronic PE/PI, the primary endpoint was TMA-free status (defined as no platelet decrease and no requirement of PE/PI or dialysis), and it was achieved in 16 of 20 (80%) patients (in the remaining 4 patients the primary endpoint failed only because of a mild decrease of platelet count). Similarly to the previous trial, most patients (80%) achieved full normalization of hematologic values (platelets and LDH); however, improvement in renal function took longer and was observed in one-third of patients.[40] These results on renal function are consistent with the mechanism of action of eculizumab, which immediately blocks the pathogenic complement derangement (as demonstrated by hematologic values) but requires longer time to recover from end-organ damages. Based on these studies, eculizumab has been approved by European Medicines Agency (EMA) and the US Food and Drug Administration (FDA) for the treatment of aHUS, and it represents the recommended therapy for this condition irrespective of the demonstration of a causative mutation, provided that other possible diagnoses (eg, thrombotic thrombocytopenic purpura) have been excluded.[41,42] Nevertheless, a possible role of eculizumab has been suggested even for the treatment of STEC-HUS[43,44] and of other forms of HUS.[42]

Antibody-mediated hemolytic anemias

It has been hypothesized that eculizumab may be effective even for the treatment of autoimmune hemolytic anemias; so far, objective evidence is scanty and mostly limited to cold agglutinin disease (CAD). CAD is due to autoantibodies of immunoglobulin M (IgM) type, which are specific for some erythrocyte antigens (usually I, more rarely i).[45] This autoimmune disorder may be primary, appearing as a chronic or subacute hemolytic anemia, or even as acute events secondary to some infections (eg, *Mycoplasma pneumoniae*, *mononucleosis*), usually with a self-limiting course.[46,47] The peculiarity of these auto-antibodies is that they have a typical thermal range, which allows the binding to erythrocytes in the cooler peripheral circulation, and subsequent complement activation in the warmer central circulation (mainly through the classical pathway). This complement activation may lead to MAC assembly and subsequent intravascular hemolysis, but more frequently simply results in an additional opsonization by C3 fragments, which may boost erythrocyte clearance through the reticulo-endothelial system. Indeed, CAD is commonly characterized by extravascular rather than intravascular hemolysis.[46,47] Eculizumab has proven to be effective in blocking intravascular hemolysis in some cases of CAD, eventually leading to therapeutic benefit.[48,49] Given the heterogeneous disease presentation and the broad spectrum of effector mechanisms (which may play different roles according to the specificity and the thermal range of patient-specific autoantibodies), it is not surprising that large experiences supporting the use of eculizumab in this condition are lacking.

Complement activation may theoretically occur in all antibody-mediated anemias, and its actual role in disease pathophysiology may differ according to the specific conditions; for instance, MAC-mediated intravascular hemolysis is also typical of isoagglutinin-mediated hemolysis as well as of paroxysmal cold hemoglobinuria.[50] In addition, the complement cascade may contribute even to anemia due to some warm (and mixed warm/cold) autoantibodies, through both MAC-mediated hemolysis and C3-mediated extravascular hemolysis.[45] Indeed, eculizumab has been considered in some refractory, life-threatening, severe hemolytic anemia as off-label, compassionate use[51]; future studies are needed to better understand the possible role of eculizumab in these specific conditions.

NOVEL COMPLEMENT INHIBITORS
Rationale for Developing Novel Anticomplement Agents

The lesson from this first decade of anticomplement treatment with eculizumab is that therapeutic complement inhibition is possible and safe and may result in substantial clinical benefit in several conditions, such as PNH and aHUS. However, this new treatment carries novel pathogenic observations as well as possible pitfalls that may limit the benefit of current treatment. In the case of eculizumab, such pitfalls are not related to the drug itself, but rather mechanistically to its effect on C5. Indeed, C3-mediated extravascular hemolysis is an obvious unmet clinical need that is emerging in PNH (together with the rare genetic resistance to eculizumab), and it paves the way for the development of novel strategies of complement inhibition and/or modulation. Later discussion describes novel complement inhibitors, which are currently in their preclinical or clinical development.[5,6] Novel complement therapeutics are categorized according to their targets and level of interception in the complement cascade, possibly anticipating their therapeutic effect in candidate clinical indications. The most relevant publically disclosed compounds are listed in **Table 1**; the specific targets and the status of development are included. A poor distinction among complement inhibitors distinguishes between agents that inhibit the effector complement and agents that are able to prevent the arming of early complement activation. C5 and C3 are the key molecules that one may wish to target to inhibit terminal effector complement or early complement activation, respectively. The interception of complement activation at the level of C3 may also exploit inhibition of the specific complement activation pathways, namely, alternative, classical, and mannose pathways.

Table 1
Candidate complement inhibitors in development for paroxysmal nocturnal hemoglobinuria and other complement-mediated diseases

Target	Name	Company	Class of Molecule	Status of Development	Ref.
C5	LFG316	Novartis/Morphosys	Monoclonal antibody	Clinical (phase II, AMD)	53
C5	Mubodina	Adienne	Monoclonal antibody (minibody)	Preclinical (non-PNH)	54,55
C5	Coversin (OmCl)	Volution Immuno-Pharmaceuticals	Small animal protein (recombinant)	Preclinical (PNH); clinical (phase I, healthy volunteers)	60
C5 (+C3?)	ATA	NA	Chemical	Preclinical (PNH)	70
C5	ARC1005	Novo Nordisk	Aptamers	Preclinical (non-PNH); clinical (phase I, AMD)	62,63
C5	SOMAmers	SomaLogic	Aptamers (SELEX)	Preclinical (non-PNH)	62,64
C5	SOBI002	Swedish Orphan Biovitrum (Affibody)	Affibody (fused with albumin-binding domain)	Preclinical (non-PNH); clinical (phase I, healthy volunteers)	62,66,67
C5	RA101348	Rapharma	Small molecule (unnatural peptide)	Preclinical (unknown)	68 (Ricardo A, Arata M, DeMarco S, et al: Development of RA101348, a potent cyclic peptide inhibitor of C5 for complement-mediated diseases. American Society of Hematology meeting 2014. Submitted for publication)
C5	Anti-C5 siRNA	Alnylam	Si-RNA	Preclinical (non-PNH and PNH)	69
C3 (C3b/iC3b)	H17	EluSys Therapeutics	Monoclonal antibody	Preclinical (PNH and non-PNH)	80,81
C3/C3b	4(1MeW)/POT-4	Potentia	Compstatin family	Preclinical (non-PNH); clinical (phase I and II, AMD)	73
C3/C3b	4(1MeW)/APL-1, APL-2	Apellis	Compstatin family	Preclinical (PNH and non-PNH); clinical (PNH and non-PNH, phase I)	78,79

Target	Agent	Company	Type/family	Status	Reference
C3/C3b	Cp40/AMY-101, PEG-Cp40	Amyndas	Compstatin family	Preclinical (PNH and non-PNH); clinical (PNH and non-PNH, planned)	77
CAP C3 convertase	TT30 (CR2/CFH)	Alexion	CFH-based protein	Preclinical (PNH and non-PNH); clinical (phase I, PNH)	92–94
CAP C3 convertase	Mini-CFH	Amyndas	CFH-based protein	Preclinical (PNH and non-PNH)	95
CAP C3 convertase	Mini-CFH	NA	CFH-based protein	Preclinical (non-PNH)	96
CAP C3 convertase	CRIg/CFH	NA	CFH-based protein	Preclinical	97
CAP and CP C3 convertase	sCR1 (CDX-1135)	Celldex	CR1-based protein	Preclinical (non-PNH); clinical (phase I, DDD)	103–105
CAP and CCP C3 convertase	Mirococept (APT070)	NA	CR1-based protein	Preclinical (non-PNH); clinical (phase I, kidney transplantation)	107–110
CAP and CCP C3 convertase	TT32 (CR2/CR1)	Alexion Pharmaceuticals	CR1-based protein	Preclinical (non-PNH)	111
CFB	TA106	Alexion Pharmaceuticals	Monoclonal antibody	Preclinical (unknown)	82
CFD	FCFD4514S	Genentech/Roche	Monoclonal antibody	Preclinical (non-PNH); clinical (phase II, AMD)	83
CFB	Anti-FB siRNA	Alnylam	Si-RNA	Preclinical (non-PNH)	69
CFB and CFD	SOMAmers	SomaLogic	Aptamers (SELEX)	Preclinical (non-PNH)	64
CFB and CFD	NA	Novartis	Small molecules (chemicals)	Preclinical (non-PNH)	86,87
Properdin	NA	Novelmed	Monoclonal antibody (and mAb derivatives)	Preclinical (unknown)	84,85
C1r/C1s	Cynryze	ViroPharma/Baxter	Human purified protein (C1-INH)	Clinical (approved for HAE)	7,90
C1s	TNT003	True North Therapeutics	Monoclonal antibody	Preclinical (Ab-mediated hemolytic anemias)	88
MASP-3	NA	Omeros	NA	Preclinical (PNH and non-PNH)	89

Abbreviation: NA, not available.

Inhibitors of Terminal Effector Complement

The inhibition of the terminal effector complement has been proven safe and effective by the anti-C5 mAb eculizumab. Thus, the interception of complement cascade preventing the cleavage of C5 by the C5 convertase represents an obvious strategy that can be exploited by novel anticomplement agents.

Antibody-based C5 inhibitors

LFG316 Two additional anti-C5 monoclonal antibodies are currently in clinical or preclinical development: LFG316 (Morphosys) is a fully human combinatorial anti-C5 mAb, which is in clinical development for AMD and other ophthalmologic diseases. After initial testing by local administration, the agent is now in phase II as systemic therapy by intravenous injection (NCT01624636).[52]

Mubodina An additional candidate agent is Mubodina, an anti-C5 "minibody," consisting of an engineered antibody fragment including only the antigen-specific variable light (VL) and heavy (VH) chain domains of its parental anti-C5 mAb.[53,54] The minibody Mubodina prevents the cleavage of C5 and inhibits the generation of inflammatory molecule C5a and of C5b, and the subsequent lytic MAC.[55] Mubodina has been approved as an orphan drug for some kidney diseases by both the FDA and EMA, and its pharmacologic inhibition of C5 cleavage (and thus of generation of C5a and C5b, and subsequently of MAC assembly[55]) anticipates an effective complement inhibition in vivo. Further derivatives of the original anti-C5 scFv are currently under development, investigating the possibility of targeting the anti-C5 agent at specific sites; this strategy, which exploits anti-C5 scFv fused with specific tag peptides, has proven effective in an animal model of arthritis[56] and might be translated in clinical application in the near future. These antibody-based inhibitors of C5 seem a ready-to-go therapeutic alternative for the rare PNH patients harboring C5 mutations, resulting in intrinsic resistance to eculizumab,[29] because the specific mutation occurs in the C5 epitope recognized by eculizumab and does not affect the binding to other antibodies.

Coversin

Another novel candidate complement inhibitor is coversin (also known as OmCI), a small (16 kDa) protein of the lipocalin family isolated from the tick *Ornithodoros moubata*.[57] Coversin binds to human C5 and prevents its cleavage by C5 convertases[58,59]; it also exerts a broader anti-inflammatory effect by binding to leukotriene B4.[58,59] Preliminary in vitro data in PNH suggest possible inhibitory effects on intravascular hemolysis as well as some effect in preventing C3 opsonization (this latter effect is not entirely clear, because it is not expected for a compound acting downstream in the complement cascade at the level of C5).[60] However, coversin has shown amenable pharmacokinetic and pharmacodynamic profiles in a phase I study in healthy volunteers following subcutaneous administration; a clinical translation plan for PNH patients is planned.[60]

Next-generation targeted C5 inhibitors

The spectrum of C5 inhibitors also includes several novel classes of compounds exploiting new technologies for specific design of more specific targeted therapeutics.

Aptamers Aptamers are large (either oligonucleic or peptide) compounds that selectively bind to specific molecules, eventually impairing their function.[61] They are usually created by using large random sequence pools, from where target-specific molecules are selected. ARC 1905 (Zimura) is a PEGylated, stabilized oligonucleic aptamer targeting C5,[62] which is currently in phase II clinical investigation for ophthalmologic disease (AMD).[63]

SOMAmers A further evolution of aptamers exploits a systematic evolution of ligands by exponential enrichment (SELEX); SOMAmers (slow off-rate modified aptamers) are these novel class of compounds with a more favorable pharmacokinetic (PK) and pharmacodynamic (PD) profile. SOMAmers specific for different key components of the complement cascade (C5, C3, complement factor D [CFD], and complement factor B [CFB]) are currently under preclinical development by SomaLogic[64] and can be considered for therapeutic application.

Affibodies A similar technology exploiting target-specific inhibition is developed by the Swedish company, Affibody, who is developing small antibody mimetic proteins (about 6 kDa) by a combinatorial protein engineering approach. The resulting small nonimmuno-globulin proteins display a high-affinity binding to a wide range of protein targets, including C5.[65] More recently, Swedish Orphan Biovitrum created a C5-specific affibody fused to an albumin-binding domain (SOBI002; 12 kDa); SOBI002 binds human C5 with low-nanomolar affinity (dissociation constant [KD] ~ 1 nM), eventually preventing its cleavage and thus the activation of the downstream effector complement. The compound demonstrated excellent bioavailability in nonhuman primates (NHP), and the fusion with the albumin-binding moiety increases half-life and stability, resulting in a terminal half-life greater than 2 weeks.[66] SOBI002 has been shown effective in preclinical models of complement (C5)-mediated diseases, and a phase I study evaluating safety, tolerability, and PK/PD in healthy volunteers has recently started (NCT02083666).[67]

Cyclomimetics Rapharma is developing another class of compounds, which are small, cyclic, peptidelike polymers with backbone and side-chain modifications, called Cyclomimetics. Cyclomimetics, which are produced by ribosomal synthesis of unnatural peptides,[68] have beneficial properties as compared with natural peptides, including a low risk of immunogenicity (due to poor major histocompatibility complex (MHC) presentation) and increased cell permeability, stability, potency, and bioavailability (due to the structural modifications). RA101348 is the lead anti-C5 macrocyclic peptide that is currently in preclinical investigation (Ricardo A, Arata M, DeMarco S, et al: Development of RA101348, a potent cyclic peptide inhibitor of C5 for complement-mediated diseases. American Society of Hematology meeting, 2014. Submitted for publication).

siRNAs The spectrum of novel anti-C5 agents is not limited to proteins or peptides; indeed, Alnylam is developing RNA therapeutics for clinical complement inhibition, targeting liver-expressed genes such as C5.[69] Robust (>95%) silencing of C5 liver production has been achieved after subcutaneous injections of GalNAc-conjugated anti-C5 siRNA duplex; in animal models, this results in sustained and durable (recovery started 2 weeks after single-dose injection) complement inhibition as effective as 90%. This agent is currently under preclinical investigations in NHP as well as in PNH in vitro. Even if siRNA-mediated complement inhibition is an elegant and promising novel therapeutic approach, further studies are needed to confirm its clinical feasibility (and efficacy, given that residual low activity might be problematic).

Chemicals The targeted design of complement therapeutics using these novel technologies offers a broad spectrum of anti-C5 inhibitors with a highly specific inhibition; thus, they seem superior to other chemicals that may intercept C5 or other complement components. For instance, aurin tricarboxylic acid (ATA) has been reported effective in preventing hemolysis of PNH erythrocytes in vitro,[70] with also a possible unexplained effect on the C3 convertase; however, it is likely that these effects of

ATA result from a broad inhibition of proteases, which may impair the function of several unrelated proteins, not restricted to complement components. Nevertheless, the rational design of novel modified chemicals with specific effect on C5 or other components of the complement cascade is possible and currently under investigation.

Inhibitors of Early Complement Activation

The attempt to inhibit complement activation at the level of C3 is a rational strategy to improve the efficacy of current anticomplement treatment, especially in PNH. The key event in early complement activation is C3 cleavage by C3 convertases generated along one of the classical complement activating pathway (CCP), alternative (CAP), and mannose (CMP). Inhibitors of early complement activation may directly target C3 or may also prevent C3 activation, exerting their effect upstream, on pathway-specific events that eventually lead to C3 activation (**Fig. 1**; see **Table 1**).

Inhibitors of complement component 3

The key event in complement activation is the cleavage of C3 into C3a and C3b by the C3 convertases; thus, C3 is an obvious target for inhibiting early complement activation. Different strategies of C3 inhibitors are currently in development; however, they have to face the problem that C3 is a large (183 kDa) and abundant (~ 1 mg/mL)

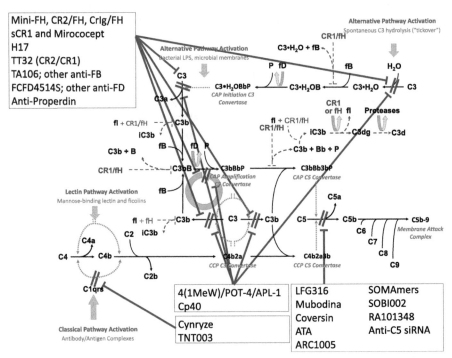

Fig. 1. Complement system and its targeted modulation. Overview of the complement cascade, including all main functional components and physiologic regulators. The 3 activating pathways (alternative, classical, and mannose/lectin) are individually depicted, together with the alternative pathway amplification loop. Candidate inhibitors are grouped according to their specific target; their modulatory effects are indicated by red lines intercepting specific steps of the complement cascade. See also main text for a more detailed description. LPS, lipopolysaccharide.

plasma protein. For this reason, it seems unlikely than anti-C3 mAbs may be used for clinical application.

Compstatin and its derivatives The use of small molecules to inhibit C3 has been pioneered by Lambris about 20 years ago with the development of a peptide named compstatin. Compstatin is a 13-residue disulfide-bridged peptide that selectively binds to human and NHP native C3 as well as to its active fragment C3b,[71] resulting in a complete inhibition of both the cleavage of C3 into C3b and the incorporation of C3b to form C3/C5 convertases.[72] Thus, compstatin prevents complement activation along all 3 complement initiating pathways (CCP, CAP, and CMP) and also inhibits the CAP amplification loop (see later discussion and **Fig. 1**), resulting in a broad and effective abrogation of all terminal effector complements (C3a, C5a, and MAC). Different compstatin derivatives[5] are currently in preclinical or clinical development: 4(1MeW) has demonstrated beneficial results in phase I clinical trials for AMD[73] and is still in clinical development by Potentia Pharmaceuticals, with the name of POT-4. The same analogue, under the name of APL-1, is developed by Appellis Pharmaceuticals for other diseases.[5] A second-generation compstatin derivative has been developed to optimize PK and PD profiles for systemic therapeutic application.[74–76] The current lead analogue, Cp40[5] (also named AMY-101), has been extensively tested in PNH in vitro.[77] Cp40/AMY-101 (and its N-terminally PEGylated derivative PEG-Cp40) demonstrated complete complement inhibition, resulting in full protection of PNH erythrocytes from MAC-mediated hemolysis[77]; furthermore, consistent with their mechanism of action, these compstatin derivatives also prevented deposition of C3 fragments on surviving PNH erythrocytes.[77] These findings provide strong evidence that the compstatin family effectively intercepts early complement activation, anticipating a clinical effect on both intravascular (MAC-mediated) and extravascular (C3-mediated) hemolysis in PNH. Indeed, these preclinical data suggest a potential therapeutic benefit over standard anti-C5 treatment; for this reason, medicine agencies from both Europe (EMA) and the United States (FDA) recently granted Orphan Drug designation to AMY-101 (ie, the Cp40-based therapeutic) for the treatment of PNH. In vivo studies of systemic administration in NHP demonstrated excellent plasma stability and favorable PK profile, with plasma half-life longer than that usually seen with other peptide drugs,[75] which may reach 5 to 6 days when using PEG-Cp40 by subcutaneous injections. These preclinical studies also showed that even unmodified Cp40/ AMY-101 has an excellent bioavailability after repeated subcutaneous injections into NHP (the terminal half-life is estimated as ∼12 hours), eventually resulting in sustained inhibitory levels with bi-daily (and possibly even daily) multidose treatment schedules.[77] Amyndas is currently starting a clinical translation plan with Cp40/AMY-101; the choice of the unmodified peptide is due to safety concerns, given that a compound with shortened half-life may allow a quicker restoration of complement activity in the case of infectious complications or other side effects. That member of the compstatin family represents an excellent candidate for clinical development in PNH and is also confirmed by data coming from another group, which has tested in vitro in PNH one first-generation analogue (APL-1) and its long-acting derivative APL-2.[78] Apellis Pharmaceuticals is currently working on a clinical trial plan (NCT02264639).[79]

Next-generation C3 inhibitors As described for C5 inhibitors, aptamers, SOMAmers, affibodies, and cyclomimetics are highly specific compounds generated by novel technologies; however, at the moment, this application remains conceptual and there are no available data, because even specific anti-C3 agents have not been disclosed yet.

Pathway-specific inhibitors
The key event of complement activation, namely, C3 cleavage, may occur along 3 distinct complement activating pathways; each of the initiating pathways (CCP, CAP, and CMP) independently leads to full activation of the complement cascade. Because each complement pathway exploits specific complement components that finally lead to C3 activation, it is theoretically possible to specifically target one complement pathway. This strategy may be particularly useful in diseases wherein the underlying pathophysiology is obviously mediated by a specific complement pathway; for example, CAP in PNH, or CCP in antibody-mediated hemolytic anemias. However, it must be acknowledged that there is also a cross-talk among the 3 complement pathways, because components of the CAP usually work to amplify the initial complement activation irrespective of the initial trigger (see **Fig. 1**).

Alternative pathway CFB and CFD are the key molecules of the activation along the CAP. CFB is a single-chain plasma protein that binds $C3(H_2O)$ generated from the spontaneous cleavage of the thioester bond of C3 (the so-called C3 tickover); after this binding, it becomes susceptible to the cleavage by CFD, which yields the noncatalytic chain Ba, and the active catalytic subunit Bb. Together with $C3(H_2O)$ (or with C3b), Bb forms the active C3 convertase, which is further stabilized by properdin. This CAP C3 convertase is transformed into C5 convertase by the further addition of a C3b molecule (analogously to the formation of CCP/CMP C5 convertases). These complement components are candidate targets for a therapeutic intervention, which aims to selectively inhibit the CAP.

   Complement activating alternative pathways C3 convertase inhibitor As discussed above, anti-C3 mAbs seem a problematic approach for early complement inhibition; however, in a recent strategy aiming to target activated C3 fragments (C3b/iC3b), rather native C3 may be feasible. An anti-C3b/iC3b mAb (3E7, and its deimmunized derivative H17) has been tested in PNH in vitro, showing a complete abrogation of hemolysis as well as of C3 deposition on surviving PNH erythrocytes.[80] These mAbs selectively inhibit CAP C3 convertase (playing on its interaction with CFB), without affecting the function of the CCP; even if mechanistically intriguing, these molecules have no future for PNH, because they should provide additional opsonins, eventually worsening rather than reducing phagocyte-mediated extravascular hemolysis. Nevertheless, engineered derivatives of H17 might open a new scenario: a Fab fragment of H17 has been described[81]; it has been tested in a preclinical model of kidney diseases and might be worthy of further investigation in PNH.

   Antibody-based inhibitors of complement factor B/complement factor H/ properdin TA106 is a Fab fragment specific for CFB, which binds to its native form, preventing its cleavage by CFD; this antibody-derived inhibitor is included in Alexion's pipeline, but preclinical data are not available yet.[6,82] In contrast, an anti-CFD mAb fragment (FCFD4514S) is in clinical development by Genentech/Roche for ophthalmologic diseases; a phase II trial is currently ongoing (NCT01602120).[82,83] Finally, humanized antiproperdin mAb and antiproperdin antigen-binding portions[84,85] are currently under development by Novelmed (public data are not available).

   Next-generation inhibitors of complement factor B/ complement factor H/ properdin The most promising strategy to target CAP components exploits small molecules that specifically bind to either CFB or CFD, preventing the interaction between these 2 proteins and the cleavage of CFB operated by CFD. The development of these specific inhibitors is in its early stage. However, small inhibitors of CFB and CFD are in preclinical investigation by Novartis[86,87] as well as by SomaLogic.[64] In addition, Alnylam is trying to exploit its siRNA technology to silence FB.[69]

Classical pathway As for the CAP, the initiation of the CCP implies the interaction of several proteins, which actually lead to the cleavage of C3 into C3a and C3b (see **Fig. 1**). The formation of CCP C3 convertase starts with the binding of antigen-bound antibodies to C1q, which activates the tetramer $C1r_2s_2$. The 2 activated C1s subunits cleave C4 into C4a and C4b, which then bind to C2, stimulating its cleavage by C1s; the resulting C4b2b complex constitutes the CCP C3 convertase. Notably, C3b generated by the CCP C3 convertase may also activate the CAP, which works to sustain and to amplify the initial CCP activation. However, targeting the CCP components involved in initial activation may result in a selective inhibition of the CCP.

Anti-C1 antibodies True North Therapeutics has recently described an anti-C1s mAb that works as a selective inhibitor of the CCP. TNT003 is a mouse IgG2a mAb that binds to C1s, thereby inhibiting its catalytic effect on C4. This compound has been investigated in vitro in CAD as a model of purely antibody-mediated hemolytic anemia.[88] TNT003 has proven effective in preventing antibody-mediated surface complement activation, preventing direct complement-mediated hemolysis triggered by the agglutinins, as well as C3 decoration of target erythrocytes.[88] TNT003 recapitulates in a CCP-mediated disease the in vitro observations seen using anti-C3 agents in PNH. Indeed, by blocking the very initial step of CCP activation, TNT003 may prevent the following: (1) C3 opsonization and subsequent C3-mediated extravascular hemolysis (which in CAD is the dominant pathogenic mechanism); (2) possible MAC-mediated intravascular hemolysis (which in CAD and other autoimmune anemias plays a minimal role due to the presence of CD55 on normal erythrocytes).[88] TNT003 is a very promising agent to be investigated in antibody-mediated anemias; indeed, even if it does not affect antibody (Ab) binding to erythrocytes (and possible fragment crystallizable (Fc) region mediated extravascular hemolysis), TNT003 may intercept complement activation that (according to the type of Ab) may contribute to the pathophysiology of hemolysis. Although hemolytic anemias mediated by Ab able to fully activate the complement (ie, IgM) seem the best indication for this agent, PNH likely would not benefit from this approach (given that Ab and CCP are not involved in its pathophysiology).

Mannose/lectin pathway The actual role of the complement mannose/lectin pathway (CMP) in human pathophysiology is not entirely elucidated; however, recent data suggest that it can be more relevant than initially thought, because of its cross-talk with the other complement pathways CCP and CAP. In the CMP, some proteins called mannose-binding lectin-associated serine proteases (MASPs, which are similar to C1r and C1s) are able to cleave C4. Mannan-binding lectin (also called mannose-binding protein), collectin, and ficolins may trigger different MASPs (MASP-1, MASP-2, and MASP-3), whereas MASP-2 are involved in activation of the CCP, MASP-3 seem relevant for the proper functioning of the AP. The availability of selective MASP inhibitors (under development by Omeros)[89] is triggering the interest for their use as novel candidate complement inhibitors.

Regulators of complement activation-based inhibitors
The development of novel complement therapeutics may exploit some physiologic regulators of complement activation (RCAs), which modulate one or more complement activation pathways; they include C1 esterase inhibitor (C1-INH), CFH, and CR1.

C1 esterase inhibitor C1-INH is a serine protease inhibitor with a broad inhibitory activity in the complement, contact, and coagulation pathways. C1-INH binds to C1r and C1s, preventing their catalytic effect on C4 and C2; this inhibitory effect on the CCP is paralleled by a similar action on the CMP, exerted via the MASPs. Constitutional deficiency or dysfunction of endogenous C1-INH results in uncontrolled complement activation, leading to hereditary angio-edema (HAE). Cinryze is a nanofiltered human plasma-derived C1-INH that is the second complement inhibitor approved for clinical use; at the moment, the only indication for Cinryze is substitutive therapy in patients with HAE.[7] Recently, Cinryze has been tested in vitro for PNH, showing a potential effect in preventing hemolysis and C3 fragment decoration of PNH erythrocytes[90]; this finding is somehow surprising, given that it should not exert any direct effect on the CAP. Whether Cinryze may play a role in the control of hemolysis in PNH or in other hemolytic anemias, it requires further mechanistic studies. In addition, its use in hemolytic conditions may require doses that are not achievable in vivo.[90]

Complement factor H-based inhibitors CFH prevents the formation of the CAP C3 convertase and accelerates its decay[91]; in addition, CFH also contributes to the inactivation of armed C3b into its inactivated form, iC3, working as a cofactor of CFI.[2] Thus, CFH has a pleomorphic role in the regulation of the CAP. Different strategies exploit its complement regulatory effect in therapeutic intervention, aiming to target it at sites of complement activation by engineered CFH-based recombinant proteins. TT30 is a 65-kDa engineered protein consisting of the iC3b/C3dg-binding domain of complement receptor 2 (CR2) fused with the inhibitory domain of CFH.[92] TT30 has been tested in vitro in PNH, demonstrating a complete inhibition of MAC-mediated intravascular hemolysis as well as a full prevention of C3 fragment deposition on surviving PNH erythrocytes.[93] The inhibitory effect of TT30 was dose-dependent and required an efficient membrane-targeting on erythrocyte surface (anti-CR2 mAb impairing TT30 binding to C3 resulted in partial reversion of the inhibitory effect).[93] These observations anticipate that TT30 should inhibit MAC-mediated intravascular hemolysis typical of PNH and may also prevent C3-mediated extravascular hemolysis, eventually emerging during anti-C5 therapies. A phase I clinical trial evaluating TT30 in PNH has just been completed (NCT01335165)[94]; the results are currently pending.

Another surface-targeted CFH-based engineered protein exploits an engineered miniaturized version of CFH (mini-CFH). Mini-CFH is a small (43 kDa) protein consisting of the regulatory complement control protein (CCP) 1–4 domains of CFH attached to its CCP 19–20 domains (which harbor a C3 binding site).[95] Indeed, mini-CFH delivers the CAP inhibitory effect of CFH (C3 convertase decay and cofactor activities) at sites of complement activation.[95] Once investigated in PNH in vitro, results were overlapping to those observed with TT30: mini-CFH effectively inhibited intravascular hemolysis of PNH erythrocytes as well as their opsonization by C3 fragments.[95] Complete CAP inhibition was achieved with mini-CFH at concentration about 10-fold lower than those seen with TT30.[95] Thus, mini-CFH (and another miniaturized version of FH[96]) is a potential candidate for treating PNH. The list of CFH-based engineered protein should be completed by another fusion protein, which exploits the complement receptor of the immunoglobulin superfamily (CRIg) as the targeting module.[97]

Complement receptor 1-based inhibitors Although CFH exerts its inhibitory role only on the CAP, CR1 is another RCA that modulates C3 activation along all 3 complement pathways[98–100]; like CFH, CR1 works as a cofactor of CFI for C3 inactivation. It exerts a direct effect on the decay of C3 and C5 convertases, which is not limited to the CAP because it also binds C3b and C4b included in the convertases of the CCP.[101] The possible role of CR1 in PNH has recently emerged with the observation that patients carrying a hypofunctional polymorphism of CR1 have a lower chance of good clinical response to eculizumab in vivo.[33] This observation was corroborated by robust in vitro data, showing that, once exposed to complement activation in the presence of C5 inhibition, PNH erythrocytes carrying the hypomorphic CR1 allele exhibited a faster and increased surface deposition of C3 fragments.[33] Furthermore, the there was an obvious quantitative effect, because erythrocytes from patients homozygous for the hypomorphic allele showed an even greater C3 opsonization,[33] clearly supporting the concept that the density of CR1 modulates complement activation and C3 deposition on PNH erythrocytes (this effect may become evident just because of the lack of CD55).

Different attempts are currently ongoing, aiming to develop CR1-based complement inhibitors.[102] A soluble CR1 (sCR1, TP10) named CDX-1135 is currently under development by Celldex; this compound has demonstrated in vitro a complete inhibition of both early (C3 convertase) and late (C5 convertase) complement activation along CCP, CAP, and CMP. CDX-1135 has been already evaluated in more than 500 patients in different clinical trials, which have confirmed its complement inhibitory effect in vivo, with negligible safety concerns. A pilot study with CDX-1135 has been initiated to explore its potential clinical benefit in patients with early-stage dense deposit disease (DDD), a kidney disorder whereby C3 consumption and deposition play an important role in disease progression (NCT01791686).[103] Preclinical data from a mouse model of DDD demonstrated that CDX-1135 may prevent the C3-mediated damage of the glomerular basement membranes[104]; furthermore, short-term compassionate use of CDX-1135 in a pediatric patient with end-stage DDD demonstrated its safety and ability to normalize activity of the terminal complement pathway.[105] Another candidate CR1-based protein is mirococept (APT070),[106] an engineered molecule consisting of the first 3 short consensus domains of CR1, attached to an amphiphilic peptide (consisting of a basic peptide and a myristoyl fatty acid group), which favors it binding to cell membranes.[107] Mirococept has been demonstrated effective in preventing complement-mediated ischemia/reperfusion injury of transplanted kidneys in rats[108] and is currently under investigation in humans in kidney transplantation.[109] A clinical randomized placebo-controlled trial investigating a method for coating the inner surface of donor kidneys with a protective layer of mirococept is ongoing, aiming to improve the function of transplanted kidneys.[110] All these CR1-based complement inhibitors (including also TT32, a CR2/CR1 fusion protein under development by Alexion)[111] represent good candidates for systemic complement inhibition in PNH and in antibody-mediated hemolytic anemias.

SUMMARY

Complement inhibition by eculizumab is effective for the treatment of PNH and other complement-mediated hemolytic anemias; however, recent data demonstrate that there is room to improve the clinical results achieved with current anticomplement agents. The spectrum of candidate complement therapeutics is growing, and different agents may entail advantages and disadvantages that may be specific for each medical condition. For instance, in PNH there is an emerging need for therapies targeting early complement activation and possible C3-mediated extravascular hemolysis. Given that the main pathogenic mechanism of hemolysis in PNH is complement activation along the CAP, one may hypothesize that broad C3 inhibitors or selective inhibitors of the CAP may be ideal for PNH. On the other hand, selective inhibitors of the CCP (such as TNT003) seem the best candidate agents for Ab-mediated hemolytic anemias such as CAD. All these strategies targeting early complement activation have to deal with a theoretic impairment of microbial defense, possibly leading to increased risk of infections that will have to be tested in vivo. The clinical development of this plethora of complement therapeutics will depend on investments done by pharmaceutical companies, which have to work in close collaboration with the scientific community; it is of extraordinary importance that the scientific community drive this development, trying to promote the development of the most promising agents in each individual disease.

REFERENCES

1. Ricklin D, Hajishengallis G, Yang K, et al. Complement: a key system for immune surveillance and homeostasis. Nat Immunol 2010;11:785–97.
2. Ricklin D, Lambris JD. Complement in immune and inflammatory disorders: pathophysiological mechanisms. J Immunol 2013;190:3831–8.
3. Pio R, Corrales L, Lambris JD. The role of complement in tumor growth. Adv Exp Med Biol 2014;772:229–62.
4. Holers VM. The spectrum of complement alternative pathway-mediated diseases. Immunol Rev 2008;223:300–16.
5. Ricklin D, Lambris JD. Complement in immune and inflammatory disorders: therapeutic interventions. J Immunol 2013;190:3839–47.
6. Ricklin D, Lambris JD. Progress and trends in complement therapeutics. Adv Exp Med Biol 2013;735:1–22.
7. Lunn M, Santos C, Craig T. Cinryze as the first approved C1 inhibitor in the USA for the treatment of hereditary angioedema: approval, efficacy and safety. J Blood Med 2010;1:163–70.
8. Risitano AM. Paroxysmal nocturnal hemoglobinuria. In: Silverberg D, editor. Anemia. Rijeka, Croatia: InTech; 2012. p. 331–74.
9. Luzzatto L, Notaro R. Paroxysmal nocturnal hemoglobinuria. In: Handin RI, Lux SE, Stossel TP, editors. Blood, principles and practice of hematology. 2nd edition. Philadelphia: Lippincot Williams & Wilkins; 2003. p. 319–34.
10. Parker CJ, Ware RE. Paroxysmal nocturnal hemoglobinuria. In: Greer J, Foerster J, Lukens J, et al, editors. Wintrobe's clinical hematology. 11th edition. Philadelphia: Lippincott Williams & Wilkins; 2003. p. 1203–21.
11. Miyata T, Takeda J, Iida Y, et al. The cloning of PIG-A, a component in the early step of GPI-anchor biosynthesis. Science 1993;259:1318–20.
12. Takeda J, Miyata T, Kawagoe K, et al. Deficiency of the GPI anchor caused by a somatic mutation of the PIG-A gene in paroxysmal nocturnal hemoglobinuria. Cell 1993;73:703–11.
13. Nicholson-Weller A, Burge J, Fearon DT, et al. Isolation of a human erythrocyte membrane glycoprotein with decay-accelerating activity for C3 convertases of the complement system. J Immunol 1982;129(1):184–9.
14. Nicholson-Weller A. Decay accelerating factor (CD55). Curr Top Microbiol Immunol 1992;178:7–30.
15. Holguin MH, Fredrick LR, Bernshaw NJ, et al. Isolation and characterization of a membrane protein from normal human erythrocytes that inhibits reactive lysis of the erythrocytes of paroxysmal nocturnal hemoglobinuria. J Clin Invest 1989;84:7–17.
16. Meri S, Morgan BP, Davies A, et al. Human protectin (CD59), an 18,000–20,000 MW complement lysis restricting factor, inhibits C5b-8 catalysed insertion of C9 into lipid bilayers. Immunology 1990;71(1):1–9.

17. Rother RP, Rollins SA, Mojcik CF, et al. Discovery and development of the complement inhibitor eculizumab for the treatment of paroxysmal nocturnal hemoglobinuria. Nat Biotechnol 2007;25:1256–64.
18. Hillmen P, Young NS, Schubert J, et al. The complement inhibitor eculizumab in paroxysmal nocturnal hemoglobinuria. N Engl J Med 2006;355:1233–43.
19. Brodsky RA, Young NS, Antonioli E, et al. Multicenter phase III study of the complement inhibitor eculizumab for the treatment of patients with paroxysmal nocturnal hemoglobinuria. Blood 2008;114:1840–7.
20. Hillmen P, Muus P, Duhrsen U, et al. Effect of the complement inhibitor eculizumab on thromboembolism in patients with paroxysmal nocturnal hemoglobinuria. Blood 2007;110:4123–8.
21. Rother RP, Bell L, Hillmen P, et al. The clinical sequelae of intravascular hemolysis and extracellular plasma hemoglobin: a novel mechanism of human disease. JAMA 2005;293:1653–62.
22. Helley D, de Latour RP, Porcher R, et al, French Society of Hematology. Evaluation of hemostasis and endothelial function in patients with paroxysmal nocturnal hemoglobinuria receiving eculizumab. Haematologica 2010;95:574–81.
23. Weitz IC, Razavi P, Rochanda L, et al. Eculizumab therapy results in rapid and sustained decreases in markers of thrombin generation and inflammation in patients with PNH independent of its effects on hemolysis and microparticle formation. Thromb Res 2012;130(3):361–8.
24. Kelly RJ, Hill A, Arnold LM, et al. Long-term treatment with eculizumab in paroxysmal nocturnal hemoglobinuria: sustained efficacy and improved survival. Blood 2011;117:6786–92.
25. Risitano AM, Notaro R, Marando L, et al. Complement fraction 3 binding on erythrocytes as additional mechanism of disease in paroxysmal nocturnal hemoglobinuria patients treated by eculizumab. Blood 2009;113:4094–100.
26. Hill A, Rother RP, Arnold L, et al. Eculizumab prevents intravascular hemolysis in patients with paroxysmal nocturnal hemoglobinuria and unmasks low-level extravascular hemolysis occurring through C3 opsonization. Haematologica 2010;95:567–73.
27. Marotta S, Giagnuolo G, Basile S, et al. Excellent outcome of concomitant intensive immunosuppression and eculizumab in aplastic anemia/paroxysmal nocturnal hemoglobinuria syndrome. J Hematol Thromb Dis 2014;2(1):128.
28. Hillmen P, Muus P, Roth A, et al. Long-term safety and efficacy of sustained eculizumab treatment in patients with paroxysmal nocturnal haemoglobinuria. Br J Haematol 2013;162(1):62–73.
29. Nishimura J, Yamamoto M, Hayashi S, et al. Genetic variants in C5 and poor response to eculizumab. N Engl J Med 2014;370(7):632–9.
30. Luzzatto L, Risitano AM, Notaro R. Paroxysmal nocturnal hemoglobinuria and eculizumab. Haematologica 2010;95(4):523–6.
31. Risitano AM, Marando L, Seneca E, et al. Hemoglobin normalization after splenectomy in a paroxysmal nocturnal hemoglobinuria patient treated by eculizumab. Blood 2008;112(2):449–51.
32. Risitano AM, Notaro R, Luzzatto L, et al. Paroxysmal nocturnal hemoglobinuria–hemolysis before and after eculizumab. N Engl J Med 2010;363(23):2270–2.
33. Rondelli T, Risitano AM, Peffault de Latour LR, et al. Polymorphism of the complement receptor 1 gene correlates with the hematologic response to eculizumab in patients with paroxysmal nocturnal hemoglobinuria. Haematologica 2014;99(2):262–6.

34. Noris M, Remuzzi G. Atypical hemolytic-uremic syndrome. N Engl J Med 2009; 361:1676–87.
35. Loirat C, Frémeaux-Bacchi V. Atypical hemolytic uremic syndrome. Orphanet J Rare Dis 2011;6:60–89.
36. Kavanagh D, Richards A, Atkinson J. Complement regulatory genes and hemolytic uremic syndromes. Annu Rev Med 2008;59:293–309.
37. Kavanagh D, Goodship T. Genetics and complement in atypical HUS. Pediatr Nephrol 2010;25:2431–42.
38. Fan X, Yoshida Y, Honda S, et al. Analysis of genetic and predisposing factors in Japanese patients with atypical hemolytic uremic syndrome. Mol Immunol 2013; 54(2):238–46.
39. Fremeaux-Bacchi V, Fakhouri F, Garnier A, et al. Genetics and outcome of atypical hemolytic uremic syndrome: a nationwide French series comparing children and adults. Clin J Am Soc Nephrol 2013;8(4):554–62.
40. Legendre CM, Licht C, Muus P, et al. Terminal complement inhibitor eculizumab in atypical hemolytic-uremic syndrome. N Engl J Med 2013;368(23): 2169–81.
41. Cataland SR, Wu HM. How I treat: the clinical differentiation and initial treatment of adult patients with atypical hemolytic uremic syndrome. Blood 2014;123(16): 2478–84.
42. Zuber J, Fakhouri F, Roumenina LT, et al, French Study Group for aHUS/C3G. Use of eculizumab for atypical haemolytic uraemic syndrome and C3 glomerulopathies. Nat Rev Nephrol 2012;8(11):643–57.
43. Orth-Höller D, Riedl M, Würzner R. Inhibition of terminal complement activation in severe Shiga toxin-associated HUS - perfect example for a fast track from bench to bedside. EMBO Mol Med 2011;3:617–9.
44. Trachtman H, Austin C, Lewinski M, et al. Renal and neurological involvement in typical Shiga toxin-associated HUS. Nat Rev Nephrol 2012;8(11):658–69.
45. Neff AT. Autoimmune hemolytic anemias. In: Greer J, Foerster J, Lukens JN, et al, editors. Wintrobe's clinical hematology. 11th edition. Philadelphia: Lippincott Williams & Wilkins; 2003. p. 1157–82.
46. Berentsen S. How I manage cold agglutinin disease. Br J Haematol 2011; 153(3):309–17.
47. Swiecicki PL, Hegerova LT, Gertz MA. Cold agglutinin disease. Blood 2013; 122(7):1114–21.
48. Roth A, Huttmann A, Rother RP, et al. Long-term efficacy of the complement inhibitor eculizumab in cold agglutinin disease. Blood 2009;113:3885–6.
49. Roth A, Duhrsen U. Cold agglutinin disease. Eur J Haematol 2010;84:91.
50. Parker CJ. Mechanisms of immune destruction of erythrocytes. In: Greer J, Foerster J, Lukens JN, et al, editors. Wintrobe's clinical hematology. 11th edition. Philadelphia: Lippincott Williams & Wilkins; 2003. p. 1139–55.
51. Bommer M, Höchsmann B, Flegel W, et al. Successful treatment of complement mediated refractory hemolysis associated with cold and warm autoantibodies using eculizumab. Haematologica 2011;94(Suppl 2):241 [abstract: 0593].
52. ClinicalTrials.gov. A service of the U.S. National Institutes of Health. Available at: http://clinicaltrials.gov/ct2/show/NCT01624636. Accessed June 10, 2014.
53. Adienne Pharma & Biotech. 2014. Available at: http://www.adienne.com/en/rd/pipeline/mubodina®.html. Accessed April 5, 2015.
54. Marzari R, Sblattero D, Macor P, et al. The cleavage site of C5 from man and animals as a common target for neutralizing human monoclonal antibodies: in vitro and in vivo studies. Eur J Immunol 2002;32(10):2773–82.

55. Woodruff TM, Nandakumar KS, Tedesco F. Inhibiting the C5-C5a receptor axis. Mol Immunol 2011;48(14):1631–42.
56. Macor P, Durigutto P, De Maso L, et al. Treatment of experimental arthritis by targeting synovial endothelium with a neutralizing recombinant antibody to C5. Arthritis Rheum 2012;64(8):2559–67.
57. Nunn MA, Sharma A, Paesen GC, et al. Complement inhibitor of C5 activation from the soft tick Ornithodoros moubata. J Immunol 2005;174(4):2084–91.
58. Roversi P, Lissina O, Johnson S, et al. The structure of OMCI, a novel lipocalin inhibitor of the complement system. J Mol Biol 2007;369(3):784–93.
59. Barratt-Due A, Thorgersen EB, Lindstad JK, et al. Ornithodoros moubata complement inhibitor is an equally effective C5 inhibitor in pigs and humans. J Immunol 2011;187(9):4913–9.
60. Weston-Davies WH, Westwood JP, Nunn M, et al. Phase I clinical trial of coversin, a novel complement C5 and LTB4 inhibitor. Paper presented at: 7th International Conference on Complement Therapeutics. Olympia, June 6–11, 2014. Aegean Conferences 82, abs 31.
61. Cox JC, Rajendran M, Riedel T, et al. Automated acquisition of aptamer sequences. Comb Chem High Throughput Screen 2002;5(4):289–99.
62. Leung E, Landa G. Update on current and future novel therapies for dry age-related macular degeneration. Expert Rev Clin Pharmacol 2013;6(5): 565–79.
63. ClinicalTrials.gov. A service of the U.S. National Institutes of Health. Available at: http://clinicaltrials.gov/ct2/show/NCT00950638. Accessed November 5, 2013.
64. Drolet DW, Zhang C, O'Connell DJ, et al. SOMAmer inhibitors of the complement system. Paper presented at: 7th International Conference on Complement Therapeutics. Olympia, June 6–11, 2014. Aegean Conferences 82, abs 23.
65. Feldwisch J, Tolmachev V. Engineering of affibody molecules for therapy and diagnostics. Methods Mol Biol 2012;899:103–26.
66. Strömberg P. Introducing SOBI002, a small Affibody-ABD fusion protein targeting complement component C5. Paper presented at: 7th International Conference on Complement Therapeutics. Olympia, June 6–11, 2014. Aegean Conferences 82, abs 30.
67. ClinicalTrials.gov. A service of the U.S. National Institutes of Health. Available at: http://clinicaltrials.gov/ct2/show/NCT02083666. Accessed November 7, 2014.
68. Josephson K, Ricardo A, Szostak JW. mRNA display: from basic principles to macrocycle drug discovery. Drug Discov Today 2014;19(4):388–99.
69. Borodovsky A, Yucius K, Sprague A, et al. Development of RNAi therapeutics targeting the complement pathway. Blood 2013;122(21):2471.
70. Lee M, Narayanan S, McGeer EG, et al. Aurin tricarboxylic acid protects against red blood cell hemolysis in patients with paroxysmal nocturnal hemoglobinemia. PLoS One 2014;9(1):e87316.
71. Sahu A, Kay BK, Lambris JD. Inhibition of human complement by a C3-binding peptide isolated from a phage-displayed random peptide library. J Immunol 1996;157(2):884–91.
72. Ricklin D, Lambris JD. Compstatin: a complement inhibitor on its way to clinical application. Adv Exp Med Biol 2008;632:273–92.
73. ClinicalTrials.gov. A service of the U.S. National Institutes of Health. Available at: http://clinicaltrials.gov/ct2/show/NCT00473928. Accessed March 16, 2010.
74. Qu H, Magotti P, Ricklin D, et al. Novel analogues of the therapeutic complement inhibitor compstatin with significantly improved affinity and potency. Mol Immunol 2011;48(4):481–9.

75. Qu H, Ricklin D, Bai H, et al. New analogs of the clinical complement inhibitor compstatin with subnanomolar affinity and enhanced pharmacokinetic properties. Immunobiology 2013;218(4):496–505.

76. Magotti P, Ricklin D, Qu H, et al. Structure-kinetic relationship analysis of the therapeutic complement inhibitor compstatin. J Mol Recognit 2009;22(6): 495–505.

77. Risitano AM, Ricklin D, Huang Y, et al. Peptide inhibitors of C3 activation as a novel strategy of complement inhibition for the treatment of paroxysmal nocturnal hemoglobinuria. Blood 2014;123(13):2094–101.

78. Kaudlay P, Hua H, He G, et al. Red cell complement loading in PNH patients on eculizumab is associated with a C3 polymorphism which influences C3 function, predicts for increased extravascular hemolysis and provides a rationale for C3 inhibition. Blood 2013;122(21):2466.

79. ClinicalTrials.gov. A service of the U.S. National Institutes of Health. Available at: http://clinicaltrials.gov/ct2/show/NCT02264639. Accessed November 25, 2014.

80. Lindorfer MA, Pawluczkowycz AW, Peek EM, et al. A novel approach to preventing the hemolysis of paroxysmal nocturnal hemoglobinuria: both complement-mediated cytolysis and C3 deposition are blocked by a monoclonal antibody specific for the alternative pathway of complement. Blood 2010;115(11): 2283–91.

81. Paixao-Cavalcante D, Torreira E, Lindorfer MA, et al. A humanized antibody that regulates the alternative pathway convertase: potential for therapy of renal disease associated with nephritic factors. J Immunol 2014;192(10): 4844–51.

82. Taube C, Thurman JM, Takeda K, et al. Factor B of the alternative complement pathway regulates development of airway hyperresponsiveness and inflammation. Proc Natl Acad Sci U S A 2006;103(21):8084–9.

83. ClinicalTrials.gov. A service of the U.S. National Institutes of Health. Available at: http://clinicaltrials.gov/ct2/show/NCT01602120. Accessed April 1, 2015.

84. Bansal R. Novelmed therapeutics. 2013. Anti-properdin antibodies. US Patent 8435512, 5 July 2013. Available at: http://www.freepatentsonline.com/8435512. html; https://www.google.com/patents/US20140186348.

85. Novelmed therapeutics. Available at: http://www.novelmed.com/ProductPipeline/ParoxysmalNocturnalHemoglobinuria(PNH).aspx. Accessed April 5, 2015.

86. Altmann E, Hommel U, Lorthiois EL, et al. Novartis Ag. Indole compounds or analogs thereof as complement factor D inhibitors useful for the treatment of age-related macular degeneration and their preparation. From PCT Int. Appl., WO 2012093101. 2012. Available at: http://www.google.com/patents/WO2012093101A1?cl=en&hl=it. Accessed July 12, 2012.

87. Dechantsreiter MA, Grob JE, Mac Sweeney A, et al. Novartis Ag. Preparation of quinazoline compounds as modulators of the complement alternative pathway for treating macular degeneration, diabetic retinopathy, and other diseases. From PCT Int. Appl., WO 2013192345. 2013. Available at: http://www.google.com.ar/patents/WO2013192345A1?cl=en&hl=it. Accessed December 27, 2013.

88. Shi J, Rose EL, Singh A, et al. TNT003, an inhibitor of the serine protease C1s, prevents complement activation induced by cold agglutinins. Blood 2014; 123(26):4015–22.

89. Scwaeble WJ. The utility of lectin pathway inhibitors as modulators if inflammatory, thrombotic and haemolytic diseases. Paper presented at: 7th International Conference on Complement Therapeutics. Olympia, June 6–11, 2014. Aegean Conferences 82, abs 25.

90. DeZern AE, Uknis M, Yuan X, et al. Complement blockade with a C1 esterase inhibitor in paroxysmal nocturnal hemoglobinuria. Exp Hematol 2014;42(10):857–61.e1.

91. Whaley K, Ruddy S. Modulation of the alternative complement pathway by β1H globulin. J Exp Med 1976;144:1147–63.

92. Fridkis-Hareli M, Storek M, Mazsaroff I, et al. Design and development of TT30, a novel C3d-targeted C3/C5 convertase inhibitor for treatment of human complement alternative pathway-mediated diseases. Blood 2011;118(17):4705–13.

93. Risitano AM, Notaro R, Pascariello C, et al. The complement receptor 2/factor H fusion protein TT30 protects paroxysmal nocturnal hemoglobinuria erythrocytes from complement-mediated hemolysis and C3 fragment. Blood 2012;119(26):6307–16.

94. ClinicalTrials.gov. A service of the U.S. National Institutes of Health. Available at: http://clinicaltrials.gov/ct2/show/NCT01335165. Accessed May 21, 2014.

95. Schmidt CQ, Bai H, Lin Z, et al. Rational engineering of a minimized immune inhibitor with unique triple-targeting properties. J Immunol 2013;190(11):5712–21.

96. Hebecker M, Alba-Domínguez M, Roumenina LT, et al. An engineered construct combining complement regulatory and surface-recognition domains represents a minimal-size functional factor H. J Immunol 2013;191(2):912–21.

97. Qiao Q, Teng X, Wang N, et al. A novel CRIg-targeted complement inhibitor protects cells from complement damage. FASEB J 2014;28:4986–99.

98. Khera R, Das N. Complement receptor 1: disease associations and therapeutic implications. Mol Immunol 2009;46(5):761–72.

99. Ross GD, Lambris JD, Cain JA, et al. Generation of three different fragments of bound C3 with purified factor I or serum. I. Requirements for factor H vs CR1 cofactor activity. J Immunol 1982;129(5):2051–60.

100. Medof ME, Nussenzweig V. Control of the function of substrate-bound C4b-C3b by the complement receptor Cr1. J Exp Med 1984;159(6):1669–85.

101. Iida K, Nussenzweig V. Complement receptor is an inhibitor of the complement cascade. J Exp Med 1981;153(5):1138–50.

102. Pratt JR, Hibbs MJ, Laver AJ, et al. Effects of complement inhibition with soluble complement receptor-1 on vascular injury and inflammation during renal allograft rejection in the rat. Am J Pathol 1996;149(6):2055–66.

103. ClinicalTrials.gov. A service of the U.S. National Institutes of Health. Available at: http://clinicaltrials.gov/ct2/show/NCT01791686. Accessed March 6, 2014.

104. Zhang Y, Nester CM, Holanda DG, et al. Soluble CR1 therapy improves complement regulation in C3 glomerulopathy. J Am Soc Nephrol 2013;24(11):1820–9.

105. Smith RJ, Xiao H, Nester CM, et al. Soluble CR1 therapy improves complement regulation in C3 glomerulopathy. Paper presented at: 7th International Conference on Complement Therapeutics, Olympia. June 6–11, 2014. Aegean Conferences 82, abs 37.

106. Souza DG, Esser D, Bradford R, et al. APT070 (Mirococept), a membrane-localised complement inhibitor, inhibits inflammatory responses that follow intestinal ischaemia and reperfusion injury. Br J Pharmacol 2005;145(8):1027–34.

107. Smith RA. Membrane-targeted complement inhibitors. Mol Immunol 2012;38:249–55.

108. Patel H, Smith RA, Sacks SH, et al. Therapeutic strategy with a membrane-localizing complement regulator to increase the number of usable donor organs after prolonged cold storage. J Am Soc Nephrol 2006;17(4):1102–11.

109. Sacks S, Karegli J, Farrar CA, et al. Targeting complement at the time of transplantation. Adv Exp Med Biol 2013;735:247–55.

110. International Standard randomised controlled trial number register. 2014. Available at: http://www.controlled-trials.com/ISRCTN49958194. Accessed August 3, 2012.

111. Holers M, Banda N, Mehta G, et al. The human complement receptor 2 (CR2)/CR1 fusion protein TT32, a targeted inhibitor of the classical and alternative pathway C3 convertase, prevents arthritis in active immunization and passive transfer models and acts by CR2-dependent targeting of CR1 regulatory activity. XXIV International Complement Workshop. Chania, October 10–5, 2012: abs #230.

Index

Note: Page numbers of article titles are in **boldface** type.

Moving?

Make sure your subscription moves with you!

To notify us of your new address, find your **Clinics Account Number** (located on your mailing label above your name), and contact customer service at:

Email: journalscustomerservice-usa@elsevier.com

800-654-2452 (subscribers in the U.S. & Canada)
314-447-8871 (subscribers outside of the U.S. & Canada)

Fax number: 314-447-8029

Elsevier Health Sciences Division
Subscription Customer Service
3251 Riverport Lane
Maryland Heights, MO 63043

*To ensure uninterrupted delivery of your subscription, please notify us at least 4 weeks in advance of move.

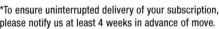
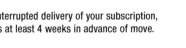

ELSEVIER

Printed and bound by CPI Group (UK) Ltd, Croydon, CR0 4YY

18/10/2024

01775941-0001